COVID-19: Origin, Impact and Management

(Part 1)

Edited by

Alfred J. Lawrence
Department of Chemistry
Isabella Thoburn College,
Lucknow, India

&

Tahmeena Khan
Department of Chemistry
Integral University,
Lucknow, India

COVID-19: Origin, Impact and Management (Part 1)

Editors: Alfred J. Lawrence & Tahmeena Khan

ISBN (Online): 978-981-5123-88-3

ISBN (Print): 978-981-5123-89-0

ISBN (Paperback): 978-981-5123-90-6

First published in 2023.

need for a court order if at any point you breach any terms of this License Agreement. In no event will any delay or failure by Bentham Science Publishers in enforcing your compliance with this License Agreement constitute a waiver of any of its rights.

3. You acknowledge that you have read this License Agreement, and agree to be bound by its terms and conditions. To the extent that any other terms and conditions presented on any website of Bentham Science Publishers conflict with, or are inconsistent with, the terms and conditions set out in this License Agreement, you acknowledge that the terms and conditions set out in this License Agreement shall prevail.

Bentham Science Publishers Pte. Ltd.
80 Robinson Road #02-00
Singapore 068898
Singapore
Email: subscriptions@benthamscience.net

BENTHAM
SCIENCE

CONTENTS

FOREWORD

The editors and authors of this book have successfully undertaken a noble and Herculean task to produce a timely guide to the coronavirus (COVID-19) pandemic that is engaging, succinct, and above all, useful to its readers. Unlike many other books about the pandemic, this book brings together experts from different fields from leading Indian and American academic institutions to provide a holistic picture of the origin, impact, and management of one of the worst pandemics humankind has ever had faced.

Such interdisciplinary thinking makes this book unique as it covers not only the science behind the origin of the virus and the development of new vaccines and drugs to fight COVID-19 and its variants but also provides us with the socioeconomic impacts of this deadly pandemic. Even though we have all been impacted by the hardship and heartbreak caused by the pandemic directly or indirectly, this book highlights the heterogeneous effect of the pandemic, particularly on developing economies and women.

I am delighted to see that each chapter in this book is devoted to a different aspect of the COVID-19 pandemic, providing the reader in a single volume with evidence-based research that will help debunk some of the misinformation and disinformation that threaten our understanding of the science behind the disease.

I do not doubt that this book will prove to be an in-depth resource for scientists, academics, researchers, students, and policymakers worldwide for years to come and help us prevent and prepare better for the next pandemic.

Dr. Arup Ganguly
The University of Mississippi (Ole Miss)
Oxford, MS, U.S.A.

PREFACE

Since the origin of the SARS-CoV-2 outbreak, the viral disease has spread like wildfire across the entire globe, hampering the quality of human life at multiple levels and causing irretrievable loss of human life. There are many aspects like psychological well-being, loss of jobs, pay cuts, loss of education and unpaid caregiving, emerging as other important consequences of the pandemic. As educators, we need to educate and provide our students with first-hand information about the ongoing crisis. This innovative book is intended to cater to scientists, academicians and students from science, humanities and commerce backgrounds to understand the pandemic from a microscopic view and how it has touched our lives at different levels. The unique special point of this book is its interdisciplinary nature making it useful for people belonging to different academic streams. A collection of topics has been explored through dedicated chapters authored by expert scientists, academicians and research scholars from leading and premier institutions. The chapters range from the very origination of the virus and factors that may facilitate its spread, like air pollution, along with the impact on nutritional, mental, psychological, and educational aspects. Mortality was not only caused by the virus, but problems like domestic violence, job cuts and suicides due to financial crunch also caused loss of lives, and these aspects are being explored by experts. The book would also provide the necessary information about the management strategies to deal with the peril caused by the COVID pandemonium. Another interesting feature of the book is the inclusion of case studies conducted with different groups like women and children to know how their lives were impacted by the pandemic and how they are coping with the situation. Another distinguishing point of the book is that the majority of the authors are women belonging to different educational backgrounds and reputed academic and research institutions. The book will prove to be of use not only to degree students and academicians but will also provide topics of interest to the common person looking to gain survey-based information on the pandemic.

Alfred J. Lawrence
Department of Chemistry
Isabella Thoburn College
Lucknow
India

&

Tahmeena Khan
Department of Chemistry
Integral University
Lucknow
India

List of Contributors

Ancey Abraham	Isabella Thoburn College, Lucknow, India
Arshi H. Khan	Integral University, Lucknow, India
Anushka Pandey	CSIR-Indian Institute of Toxicology Research (CSIR-IITR), Lucknow, India
Angila Shahab	Jamia Milia Islamia, New Delhi, India
Ayushi Tewari	District Institute of Education and Training (DIET), Lucknow, India
Anju Verma	Indian Institute of Technology, Kanpur, India
Brijesh Singh	Indian Institute of Technology, Kanpur, India
Faiza Ali	Isabella Thoburn College, Lucknow, India
Insha Abbas	Institute of Bioinformatics and Applied Biotechnology, Bangalore, India
Jagrati Sharma	Isabella Thoburn College, Lucknow, India
Mehul Raithatha	Indian Institute of Management, Indore, India
Nitya Dubey	Indian Institute of Technology, Kanpur, India
Pavan Kumar Nagar	Indian Institute of Technology, Kanpur, India
Robinson Reyes-Peña	College of Business Administration, Florida International University, Miami, FL, USA
Saima Arif	CSIR-Indian Institute of Toxicology Research (CSIR-IITR), Lucknow, India
Saimah Khan	Integral University, Lucknow, India
Saman Raza	Isabella Thoburn College, Lucknow, India
Tahmeena Khan	Integral University, Lucknow, India
Tuba Siddiqui	Integral Institute of Medical Sciences and Research, Lucknow, India

CHAPTER 1

The Outbreak of COVID-19 Coronavirus and Associated Facts and Factors

Anushka Pandey[1], **Anju Verma**[2], **Pavan Kumar Nagar**[2] and **Tahmeena Khan**[3,*]

[1] *Toxicokinetics Laboratory, CSIR- Indian Institute of Toxicology Research (IITR), Lucknow-226001, Uttar Pradesh, India*

[2] *Indian Institute of Technology, Kanpur, India*

[3] *Department of Chemistry, Integral University, Lucknow, India*

Abstract: COVID-19 is a global pandemic resulting in devastating impacts that spread through a virus and are even more contagious than influenza, as evident from the frequent reporting of cluster outbreaks. Although the key problem is that the symptoms are often similar to other common illnesses, such outbreaks can be controlled if individuals with initial symptoms are tested, and further contact tracing is done. The concept presented here discusses the order in which symptoms appear to differentiate it from other respiratory disorders, however, this crucial information is mostly missing. To determine the most likely order of detectable symptoms in COVID-19 patients, we apply a Markov Process to a graded partially ordered set based on clinical observations of COVID-19 cases. A comparison was made between the evolution of these symptoms in COVID-19 and influenza, SARS, and MERS to see if they were present differently. Influenza, according to our hypothesis, begins with a cough, whereas COVID-19 and other coronavirus infections begin with a fever. COVID-19, on the other hand, varies from SARS and MERS in terms of the order of gastrointestinal symptoms. As facilities begin to reopen following the 2020 spring outbreak, our findings support the idea that fever should be used to screen for admission and that appropriate clinical practice should include noting the order of symptoms occurrence in COVID-19 along with other diseases. If this type of systemic clinical approach had been routine, the move from a local to a worldwide pandemic might not have happened.

Keywords: Clinical approach, COVID-19, Fever, Infections, Markov Process, MERS, Pandemic, SARS, Variants.

* **Corresponding author Tahmeena Khan**: Department of Chemistry, Integral University, Lucknow, India; E-mail: tahminakhan30@yahoo.com

Alfred J. Lawrence & Tahmeena Khan (Eds.)

INTRODUCTION

COVID-19

For the initial novel coronavirus-infected pneumonia (NCIP) cases in Wuhan, Hubei Province, China, we analysed the data of the first 425 confirmed cases to determine the epidemiologic characteristics of NCIP. Most avian influenza A (H7N9) cases in mainland China during the spring of 2013 were reported by pneumonia of an unknown aetiology (PUE) surveillance system. For assessing the role of surveillance bias and possible underreporting in the assessment of the epidemiology of subtype H7N9 cases and the effects of poultry market closures, all PUE cases were analysed, which got reported from 2004 to May 3, 2013 [1].

PUE reporting was inconsistent and was biased towards A (H7N9) affected provinces. No evidence was found that the older ages of persons with A (H7N9) resulted from surveillance bias. The decline in PUE cases after poultry market closures indicates outbreak control [2].

On March 31, 2013, China reported the first human infection of the A (H7N9) virus to the WHO, and as of May 3, 2013, a total of 127 cases resulting in 24 deaths had been reported. The median age of the case patients was 62 years, with 71% of them being males [3].

The first COVID-19-reported individuals who showed symptoms as early as 8th December 2019 were among the stallholders of the Wuhan South China Seafood Market, after which it was closed down on Jan 1. After performing the gene sequencing on Jan 10, it was confirmed to be a novel coronavirus, related to the MERS-CoV and SARS-CoV however, its mortality and transmissibility are still unknown, which are likely to differ from the prior ones [4]. A detailed image of the COVID-19 virus is shown in (Fig. **1**).

People who got infected and travelled abroad are the carriers of the virus and the initiation of a global outbreak was marked. 13th January 2020 was the first internationally reported case from Thailand outside China [5].

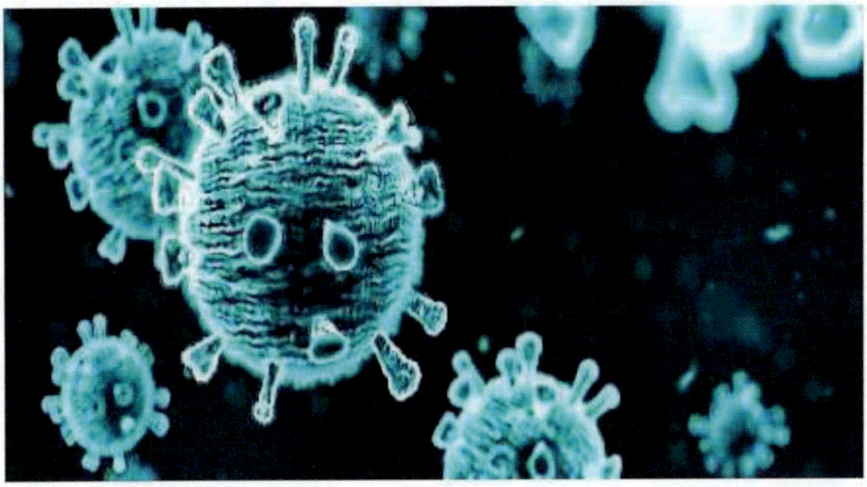

Fig. (1). Digital image of COVID-19 Virus.

On January 22, 2019, the WHO emergency committee discussed whether to declare it a public health emergency of international concern (PHEIC) under health regulations, but went undecided in the absence of full-proof information [6].

On 23rd January 2020, Wuhan suspended all public transport and air travel and placed residents under quarantine. Screening of people in public places, along with the railways and airways places, was extensively carried out globally [7].

Dashboard for Geographic Information Systems (Updated April 27, 2020)

In light of the current public health crisis, we created an interactive web-based dashboard that was hosted by John Hopkins University's Centre for System Science and Engineering (CSSE) for the visualisation and tracking of cases reported in real-time. On 22nd January 2020, it was publicly shared, illustrating the places and the number of recorded COVID cases, deaths, and recoveries, as well as their locations (Fig. **2**). This user-friendly application was created for researchers and health authorities to use as a reference tool, as well as to assist the general public in keeping track of the occurrence. Its data is publicly available and is now shown in the ESRI Living Atlas.

As the manual reporting process becomes difficult with the accelerating of cases being reported globally, we decided to embrace it. A semi-automated living data stream strategy was implemented. DXY, an online platform run by members of the Chinese medical community, was our primary data source initially, but then as time went on, we created a series of data sources which included US county and state health departments, national government health departments, and data aggregating websites like Worldometers.info, BNO, and the COVID tracking Project. The CSSE COVID-19 GitHub Repository has all of our sources, and a JHU team is responsible for data protection and revisions [8].

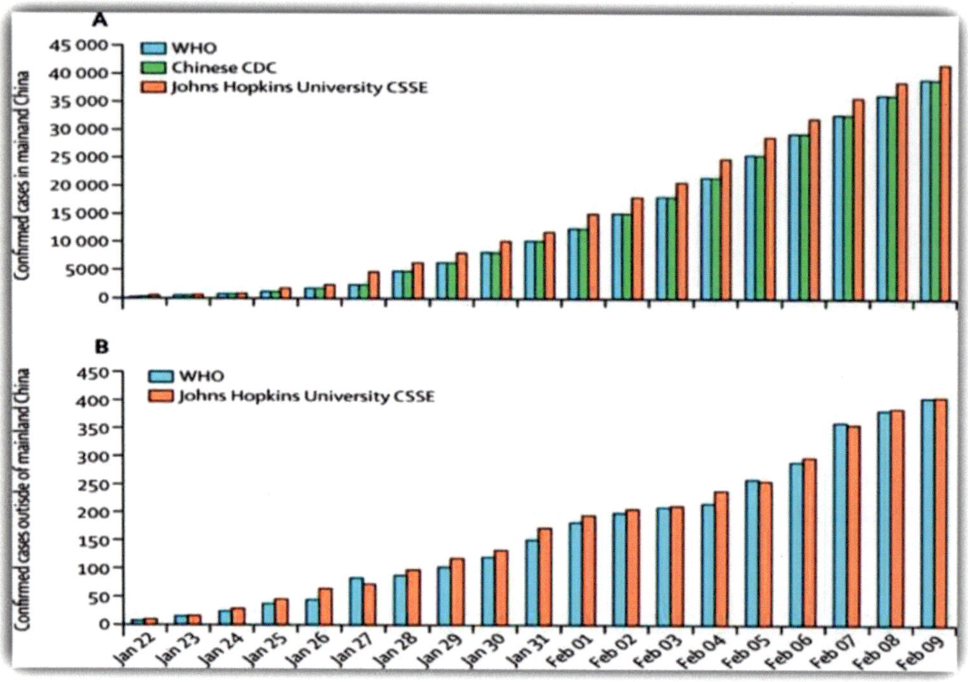

Fig. (2). Daily cumulative case numbers (starting Jan 22, 2020) reported by the Johns Hopkins University Centre for System Science and Engineering (CSSE), WHO situation reports, and the Chinese Centre for Disease Control and Prevention (Chinese CDC) for within **(A)** and outside **(B)** mainland China from different sources [8].

TYPES OF VARIANTS

Variants being monitored, variants of worry, variants of interest, and variances of utmost importance are examples of classifications. Some of them appear to spread faster and easier than others, which might also lead to an increase in COVID-19 cases, exerting more load on the medical system and potentially leading to more hospitalisation and fatalities.

Above that, the types are based on the ease with which the variant spreads, the severity of its symptoms, and how it reacts to medications and immunizations.

Variants of Concern in the India & US: Delta Variant

Delta – B.1.617.2

India was the first to report it. It spreads more quickly than other variants, as well as causing more extreme sickness.

CDC released updated guidance on the need for increasing COVID vaccination coverage and also other precautionary measures for fully vaccinated people as well on 27th July 2021 as several studies and new data keeps emerging.

After a decline from January 2021, a significant increase in cases is seen with increases in hospitalization rates around the country. The case rate looks similar to the earlier time when vaccinations weren't available. Secondly, as from recent CDC, published data and other reports signal that the Delta variant was more infectious and led to increased transmissibility even in some vaccinated individuals. Unpublished surveillance data will also be publicly available in the coming weeks.

Delta, at present, is the predominant variant in the US. As more information will come out and be made available when more data are published, studies will be conducted in the coming weeks. As of now, CDC's high-level summary is presented below from whatever scientists so far have come to know [9].

Infections and Spread

The Delta form of SARS-CoV-2 is more infectious and spreads faster than other SARS-CoV-2 strains.

- Some studies, such as that from Canada and Scotland, suggest it might lead to more severe illness than the earlier variants in unvaccinated people.
- Non-vaccinated people are more likely to become infected and spread the virus in society, posing a greater risk of transmission. CDC is monitoring regularly to assess whether fully vaccinated people being asymptomatic can transmit the virus.
- For the cases of earlier variants of COVID-19, when the viral genetic material from the samples was analysed, it was found that the lower amounts of it were found in the fully vaccinated people who got the breakthrough infections than in the unvaccinated ones. For the case of Delta, the amounts found were similar; however, unlike prior variants, the amount of viral material may go down faster in fully vaccinated ones than the unvaccinated ones [9].

Vaccine

Preliminary research shows that when fully vaccinated people are diagnosed with the Delta variant, they can transfer the virus to others. However, infections only affect a tiny percentage of people and are very successful in preventing death or severe illness.

Treatments

Almost all variants in the US responded to the treatment of FDA-authorized monoclonal antibody treatments.

Statement from the Centre for Disease Control and Prevention (CDC) on B.1.1.529 (Omicron Variant)

Identified first: South Africa

Immediate release date: 26th November 2021

WHO classified a new variant as a Variant of Concern named Omicron on 26th November 2021. US hasn't yet identified any case so far inside it though CDC is following up with this new update. Humans are thankful to the South African government and researchers for publicly reporting this to the rest of the world and continuing to share pertinent information with the US Ministry of Health Services and the Centre for Disease Control and Prevention (CDC). We'll keep you updated as we continue to track this development and collaborate with worldwide public health and industrial collaborators to learn more.

CDC recommends preventive measures that people should follow, such as wearing a mask in public places, washing or sanitizing their hands whenever necessary and maintaining physical distance from others. It is advisable to get fully vaccinated, and CDC encourages booster doses for those who are eligible and travellers should follow the proper travel advice from the Centre for Disease Control and Prevention [10].

Update

As more information becomes available, the CDC will publish updates. India has recorded 213 Omicron Cases as of December 22, 2021. India has confirmed 200 cases of Omicron as of December 21, 2021. (Coronavirus). Of 200 cases, 123 cases are active, and the remaining 77 have been discharged or recovered.

In the meantime, Omicron is spreading rapidly, and it could soon account for more than half of COVID-19 cases (2nd December 2021).

The following are the most important details to be aware of:

1. As new variants emerge, it is important to take necessary precautions to limit the transmission of infection and obtain a vaccination to slow the formation of new variants.
2. Vaccination programmes will reduce severe illness and hospitalization cases along with deaths.
3. All COVID-19 detecting tests will detect all the variants but, can't say about the infected variant in particular.

Why a booster dose of vaccine is required?

In light of the new variant's hazard, WHO recommends that those who receive entire inactivated virus-based vaccines, as well as those who are most immuno-compromised, obtain booster doses.

COVID-19 CASES IN INDIA

Between the 3rd of January 2020 and the 30th of November 2021, the WHO reported 34,587,822 confirmed cases of Covid, with 468,980 deaths. Vaccines were given out in a total of 1,183,573,646 doses until November 22nd, 2021 [6] Table **2**. Table **1** summerised the number of cases and deaths reported by the WHO in India according to different states.

Table 1. Number of cases and deaths reported by the WHO in India according to different states.

Location	Cases	Deaths
Andaman and Nicobar Islands	7,683 7,683	129 129
Andhra Pradesh	20.7L 20,70,000	14,439 14,439
Arunachal Pradesh	55,273 55,273	280 280
Assam	6.17L 6,17,000	6,098 6,098
Bihar	7.26L 7,26,000	9,663 9,663
Chandigarh	65,456 65,456	820 820
Chhattisgarh	10.1L 10,10,000	13,593 13,593
Delhi	14.4L 14,40,000	25,098 25,098

(Table 1) cont.....

Location	Cases	Deaths
Goa	1.79L 1,79,000	3,384 3,384
Gujarat	8.27L 8,27,000	10,092 10,092
Haryana	7.72L 7,72,000	10,054 10,054
Himachal Pradesh	2.27L 2,27,000	3,847 3,847
Jammu and Kashmir	3.37L 3,37,000	4,476 4,476
Jharkhand	3.49L 3,49,000	5,140 5,140
Karnataka	30L 30,00,000	38,203 38,203
Kerala	51.4L 51,40,000	39,955 39,955
Ladakh	21,540 21,540	214 214
Lakshadweep	10,394 10,394	51 51
Madhya Pradesh	7.93L 7,93,000	10,528 10,528
Maharashtra	66.3L 66,30,000	1.41L 1,41,000
Manipur	1.25L 1,25,000	1,975 1,975
Meghalaya	84,461 84,461	1,472 1,472
Mizoram	1.35L 1,35,000	493 493
Nagaland	32,109 32,109	696 696
Odisha	10.5L 10,50,000	8,409 8,409
Puducherry	1.29L 1,29,000	1,872 1,872
Punjab	6.03L 6,03,000	16,599 16,599
Rajasthan	9.55L 9,55,000	8,955 8,955

(Table 1) cont.....

Location	Cases	Deaths
Sikkim	32,233 32,233	403 403
Tamil Nadu	27.3L 27,30,000	36,472 36,472
Telangana	6.76L 6,76,000	3,990 3,990
Tripura	84,791 84,791	823 823
Uttar Pradesh	17.1L 17,10,000	22,910 22,910
Uttarakhand	3.44L 3,44,000	7,408 7,408
West Bengal	16.2L 16,20,000	19,473

MATERIALS AND PROCEDURES

Data Gathering

COVID-19 Discernible Symptoms in Possible Order

Many hospitals have been over-occupied due to an exponential increase in cases in the current pandemic. Those who have the mild form of the disease are advised to seek consultation from their home in isolation. We chose to include these four symptoms in the Stochastic Progression Model because they are similar to those of other respiratory disorders. When the odds for each symptom are uniformly random, the occurrence of symptoms associated was determined first to confirm the model's validity. The most and least likely avenues for the occurrence of the four symptoms are illustrated in the diagram below by red and blue lines, respectively. Each conceivable path is equally likely, with the least and most common pathways describing the most often and least likely set of symptoms that a randomly infected person in the population might suffer [11].

In COVID-19, the Order of Discernible Symptoms is Unrelated to the Severity of the Disease Just at the Time of Admission

We used the Stochastic Progression Model for each group of cases independently after separating the dataset of COVID-19 cases (N= 1099) into severe and non-severe patients as identified during admitting, and investigating the influence of severity on the order of observable symptoms. In both severe and non-severe cases, it was discovered that the most and least likely courses are identical. To highlight these similarities, the most significant variation in likelihood is noted when the most likely path transitions from no symptoms to fever. In severe and non-severe instances, probabilities of 0.775 and 0.818 were found, showing a difference of 0.043 (Fig. **3**). All of these findings support the idea that fever is the first symptom of COVID-19 and the order of detectable symptoms is unaffected by severity [12].

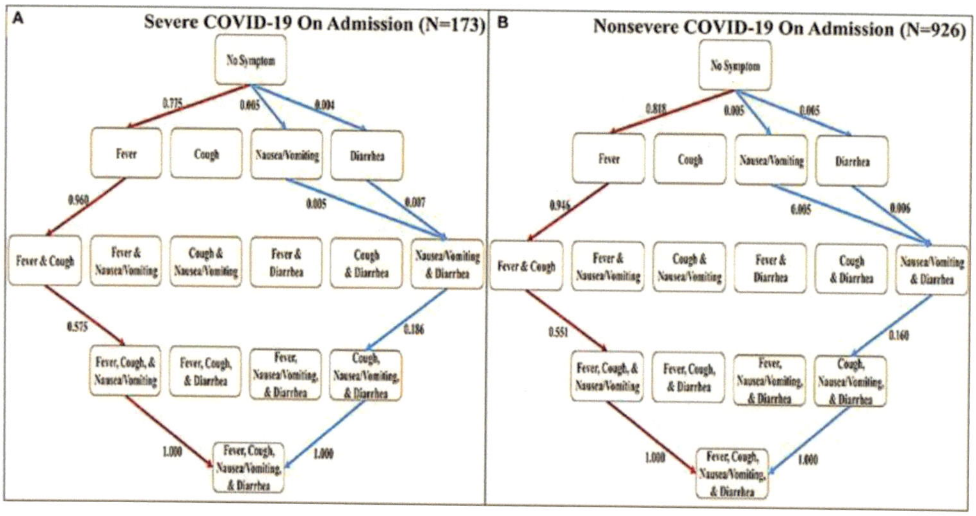

Fig. (3). Illustrates the most and least likely routes of detectable symptoms in COVID-19 instances with severe and non-severe COVID-19. **(A)** Hasse Diagram representing COVID-19's most likely (red) and least likely (blue) routes for cases classified as severe on admission based on transition probabilities reported here. **(B)** Hasse Diagram depicting most likely (red) and least likely (blue) COVID-19 routes for cases classified as non-severe on admission based on transition probabilities reported here [13].

Variation of Respiratory Disorders & the Order of Observable Symptoms

We used the Stochastic Progression Model to estimate the least and most likely routes for four respiratory diseases: COVID-19, influenza, MERS, and SARS. The four observable symptoms are objective and reasonably easy for physicians and patients to validate. Fever, cough, nausea/vomiting, and diarrhoea are the most common symptoms of COVID-19. It's identical to influenza by reversing the sequence of the first two symptoms listed above. The most likely pathways for MERS and SARS are the same, namely fever, cough, diarrhoea, and eventually nausea/vomiting (Fig. **4**).

COVID-19 and MERS have the same least likely path, although influenza is different from the other diseases [13].

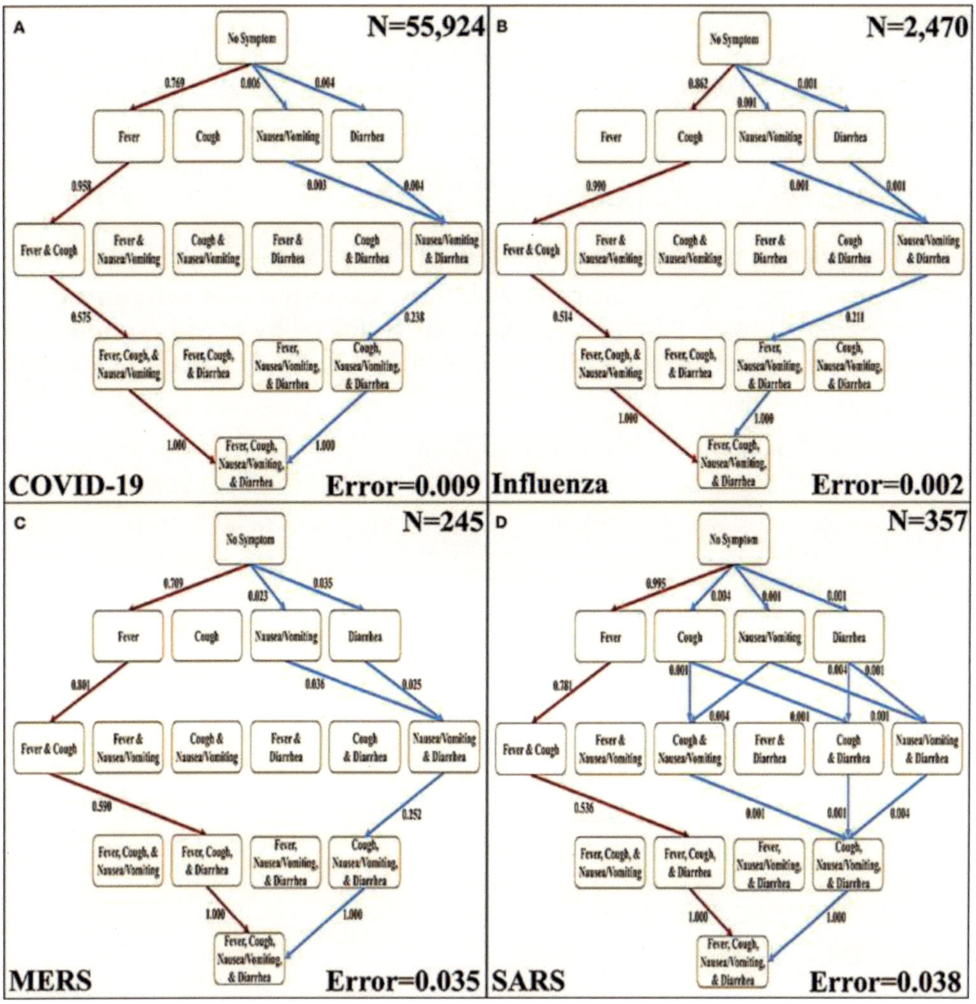

Fig. (4). The most likely and least likely pathways for detecting symptoms in respiratory disorders. **(A)** A Hasse Diagram depicting the most likely (red) and least likely (blue) routes for COVID-19 symptoms. **(B)** In a Hasse Diagram for influenza symptoms, the most likely (red) and least likely (blue) routes are shown. **(C)** In a Hasse Diagram for MERS symptoms, the most likely (red) and least likely (blue) routes are shown. **(D)** In a Hasse Diagram for SARS symptoms, the most likely (red) and least likely (blue) routes are shown. The most and least likely pathways are computed for each diagram using the transition probabilities indicated on the edges. The sample size (N) and inaccuracy of transition probabilities are also shown [13].

Using COVID-19 to Compare the Order of the Most Prevalent Symptoms in Respiratory Diseases

Due to the specific feature of most and least likely routes, active monitoring of the identifiable sequence of symptoms could be valuable, but we extended our research to the seven symptoms reported commonly in all four respiratory disorders studied here. The second group of subjective symptoms, such as sore throat, myalgia, and headache, was formed. Implementing the COVID-19's Stochastic Progression Model for the 7 symptoms yielded findings that did not disturb the original ordering, but rather introduced another level of complication in the middle of the likely paths, transitioning to fever for the most likely path and cough for the second. The difference in the likelihood of developing a sore throat, headache, or myalgia was imperceptible [14].

Despite the difficulty of implementation, it is consistent with our previous findings. The most likely course of COVID-19 was eventually determined to be fever, cough, sore throat, myalgia, or headache, followed by nausea/vomiting, and diarrhoea, which is consistent with the confirmed COVID-19 cases dataset (Fig. 5) [13].

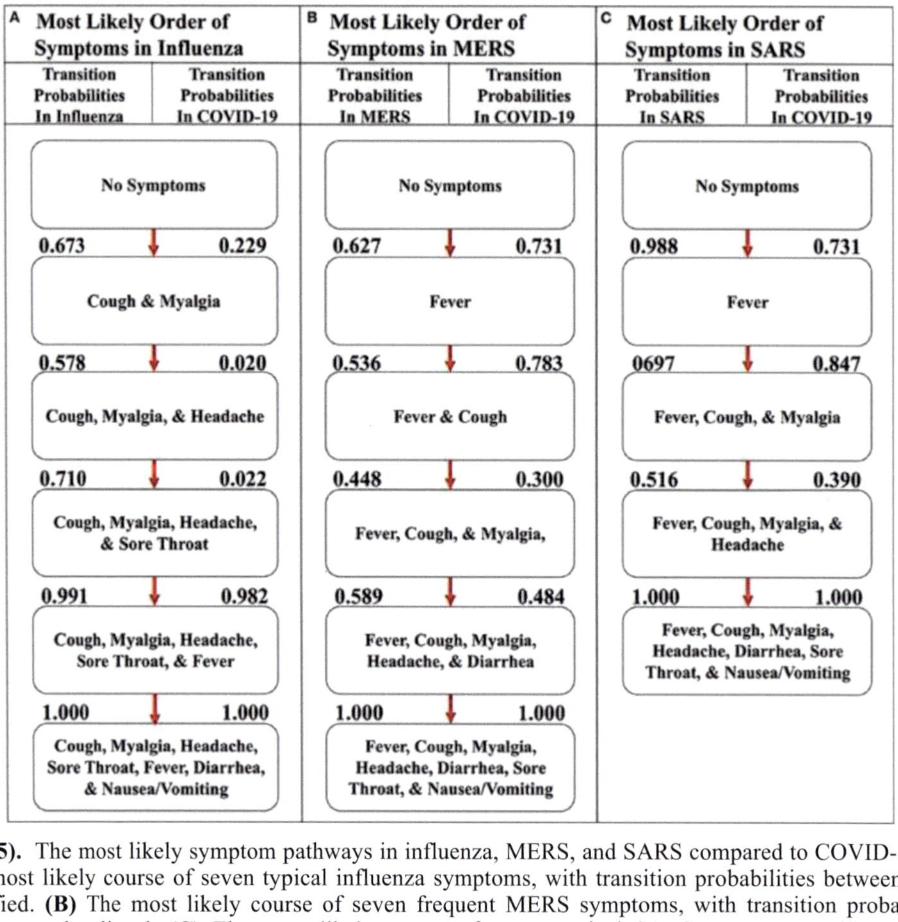

Fig. (5). The most likely symptom pathways in influenza, MERS, and SARS compared to COVID-19. **(A)** The most likely course of seven typical influenza symptoms, with transition probabilities between nodes specified. **(B)** The most likely course of seven frequent MERS symptoms, with transition probabilities between nodes listed. **(C)** The most likely course of seven typical SARS symptoms, with transition probabilities between nodes listed. The transition probabilities in COVID-19 are listed on the right for each path. The transition probabilities given between nodes on the left are used to calculate the most likely routes for each disease [13].

Various works in the area of research COVID-19 outbreak have evaluated transition probabilities for the same path in other respiratory illnesses to illustrate the uniqueness of COVID-19's most likely path. After comparing the two, we discovered that the implementation representing COVID-19 strongly suggests that fever will be the first symptom, with cough following shortly after, due to transition probabilities of 0.731 and 0.783, respectively, whereas the implementation representing influenza strongly suggests that fever will be the first symptom, with a probability of 0.035. Furthermore, with values of 0.627 and 0.988, respectively, MERS and SARS data had a considerable risk of initially changing to fever. In a similar way to fever and cough, COVID-19 and the other three diseases are associated with three subjective symptoms. These results corroborate previous research.

FACTORS AFFECTING COVID-19 OUTBREAK

Adolescents and Teenagers with Coronavirus Disease (COVID-19)

In this Globalization world and interconnected lives, it's easy for a virus to turn into an outbreak. There are numerous factors influencing the spread and transmission of it, such as population density, social & economic status, healthcare infrastructure, awareness vaccination programmes, *etc.*

COVID-19 can be caught by anyone, regardless of age. As we continue to learn more about how it affects people, studies and data as of now, suggest that children below the age of 18 years have few deaths and usually mild diseases though cases of critical illness have been reported [15].

Infected people of all ages can transmit the virus to others if they have minimal or no symptoms. It is conveyed through the nose or mouth by liquid particles such as aerosols, which are spread when an infected person coughs, sneezes, or speaks. As a result, it's best to keep a gap of at least 1 metre between yourself and others.

If one was meant to acquire HPV, meningitis, and tetanus vaccinations, but immunisation services were unavailable, then routine vaccines should be carried out as soon as possible, according to the World Health Organization. For example, the two-dose HPV vaccine can be started at any age between 9 and 14, and the time between doses can be extended. Six months is the minimum time between doses, although it can be prolonged to twelve to fifteen months or even longer if necessary.

The constant flood of news, which can be conflicting at times, can make anyone feel bewildered and stressed. To obtain information, we should rely on credible sources, such as UNICEF and WHO. For the most up-to-date information, download the WHO Health Alert app for WhatsApp.

This is a new, free-to-use service that provides timely, accurate, and official information 24 hours a day, worldwide. To get started, click the WHO Health Alert and then just text the word “Hi” in a WhatsApp message. Similar programmes exist in many nations to give context-specific information and updates. Remember that inundating yourself with information on the COVID-19 pandemic can be stressful, so look for updates and practical advice at specified times during the day and avoid listening to or following rumours that make you feel uneasy.

So far, no evidence of COVID-19 being transmitted by sperm or vaginal secretions has been found. Masturbation, on the other hand, does not put a person at risk of becoming infected if they have sex with someone who has COVID-19. To avoid STDs and unplanned pregnancies, make sure to use condoms and contraception.

Some of the things you can do to maintain your safety while at home are listed below:

- You could politely but firmly tell him that you do not want him to touch you and that he should stop.
- You could tell your parents, other caretakers, or a trustworthy adult in the house what's going on.
- You may tell a trusted adult outside your house, like a neighbour, a teacher, a family friend, or a relative.
- If you have a phone, you can call or text for assistance and support. This includes phoning a child protection service in your area or dialling a hotline/helpline for children and women who require assistance, are distressed, or have been victims of abuse. Make sure your phone calls and text messages aren't left anywhere where they could be accessed by others.
- If you need to leave the house right away because he is injuring or harming you, consider making a discreet pre-arrangement with a neighbour, trusted relative, or family friend to help you leave and stay with them until it is safe to return home.
- If you have been sexually abused or raped and require immediate medical attention, go to the nearest hospital or clinic as soon as possible.

When will this pandemic come to an end, allowing things to return to normal?

We don't know when it will end, but the combined efforts of all persons will aid in preventing the virus's spread. The implementation of nationwide lockdowns has slowed the spread of the infection in the community. It is critical and suggested that we continue to follow the COVID protocols to protect everyone's safety.

As far as we know, it existed naturally in animals before being passed on to humans. As evidenced by the increasing number of such instances during the 1980s, increased deforestation, intense farming methods, improper management, and wildlife eating increase the danger of new developing infectious diseases. Healthy wildlife and the environment are linked to human health and should be protected and cared for intelligently. The illegal trafficking of wild animals is also a serious concern.

Breastfeeding and Coronavirus

There hasn't been any proof found so far that COVID-19 is transferred through breastfeeding. Therefore this was of major concern. Should mothers breastfeed in communities where COVID-19 is prevalent? So, the answer to this is that breastfeeding benefits the growth and survival of newborn newborns, hence mothers should breastfeed. Immediate and ongoing skin-to-skin care, such as that provided by kangaroo mothers, enhances newborns' temperature management and is linked to increased survival. Placing the newborn close to the mother also allows for the early start of breastfeeding, which lowers mortality. The enormous advantages of skin-to-skin contact and nursing vastly outweigh the potential hazards of COVID-19 transmission and sickness.

When you feel healthy enough, you can begin breastfeeding. There is no set amount of time to wait after COVID-19 has been confirmed or suspected. There is no indication that breastfeeding affects a mother's COVID-19 clinical course. Healthcare professionals or lactation counsellors should assist in lactating.

- Donor human milk;
- Expressing milk

If releasing breast milk or obtaining donor human milk is not an option, try wet-nursing (when the kid is breastfed by another woman) or infant formula milk, with mechanisms in place to guarantee that it is possible, properly prepared, safe, and long-term.

As none of the licensed vaccines currently in use is a live virus, therefore there is no risk of the virus being passed through breast milk. Also, at the same time, it is seen that after vaccination, antibodies are found in breast milk, which can help protect the newborn against COVID-19 so, so women can take vaccines who are breastfeeding.

Coronavirus Disease (COVID-19): Contact Tracing

Touch tracing is when those who have been in close contact with or near those who have been infected with COVID-19 and are at risk of contracting the infection and further spreading the disease are tracked down as soon as feasible. Contact tracing is still effective against new COVID-19 viral strains and helps to break the chain of transmission through early identification, isolation and medical care of the individuals.

Individuals who are kept separated from the rest people after they are known to get in contact with the infected individuals are likely to be the carrier of the virus, whereas isolation is the separation of people who are known to be infected already with COVID-19.

Climate Science and Coronavirus Disease (COVID-19)

Although temperature and humidity may affect how long the virus persists from the outside human body or on the surface and in the air, there is no evidence that weather or climate affects the prevalence of COVID-19.

We know that air pollution is a rising global concern, and efforts have been put into mitigating the emissions of greenhouse gases. Due to lockdowns across the globe and shutdown of the majority of industries and economic activities, there have been temporary improvements in the air quality levels in some areas, but once all get open up, then these air quality levels will deteriorate back again, and this downtrend at the cost of livelihoods isn't a viable substitute in the fight against the rising pollution.

Contraception and Family Planning are Important in the Case of Coronavirus Disease (COVID-19)

During the COVID-19 epidemic, why is it vital to provide contraception/family planning, as well as family planning services and information?

Contraception and access to birth control are vital aspects of a healthy lifestyle and avoiding unplanned pregnancies and sexually transmitted infections (STIs for families. Also, due to the COVID outbreak, the health sector and medical staff are already burdened with the patient load. To stop the build-up of additional pressure from different diseases and consultations, it becomes even more important.

Coronavirus Disease (COVID-19): HIV-Positive Persons and COVID-19 Vaccinations

Although the trials for the same were conducted with a small number of HIV-positive persons, existing evidence suggests that the WHO-recommended vaccines are safest to use for HIV-positive people. Furthermore, no pharmacological interactions or interruptions between the COVID vaccination and HIV antiretroviral medicines have been recorded.

Science-based literature has recently entered the debate, causing widespread concern about a possible link discovered more than a decade ago between adenovirus vector-based vaccines and an increased risk of HIV infection in men who receive that kind of vaccine. However, the reasons for this appear to be uncertain, and many more obey studies are now being performed.

It's entirely feasible that persons with HIV who have low CD4 cell counts have a lower immune response to vaccines, but this hasn't been proven in practice for all vaccines, and there's no data to back it up. WHO will issue an update as soon as possible. To obtain more verified efficacy, it is also vital to ensure that patients living with HIV are included.

WHO advises nations to consult the WHO SAGE Roadmap For Prioritizing Uses of COVID-19 Vaccines In The Context Of Limited Supply [16], which was developed with the assumption that vaccination efficacy would be similar across subgroups (for example, in people with comorbidities that increase the risk of severe COVID-19 such as HIV-positive status). As a result, countries can plan for people to receive the vaccine in order of priority based on their age, health, occupation, and other characteristics, such as those in care or residential homes, or those in closed settings such as prisons.

Vaccination is being prioritised in several countries for all living with HIV or for those who are immunocompromised (as evidenced by a CD4 cell count of less than 200/mm^3) [17]. At least 40 countries in all regions, according to an informal poll of more than 100 countries, have an immunisation strategy that prioritises immunizations for HIV-positive people. Recent research reveals that people living with HIV, regardless of CD4 cell level, are at a higher risk of severe outcomes and death from COVID-19 when compared to people who do not have HIV [18]. Many persons living with HIV, regardless of immunological status, have one or more comorbidities that place them at higher risk for a more severe COVID-19.

HIV infection is a substantial independent risk factor for both severe/critical COVID-19 presentation at hospital admission and in-hospital death, according to a recent WHO analysis. COVID-19 hospitalisation resulted in the deaths of nearly a quarter of all HIV patients (23.1%) [19]. The report is based on clinical surveillance data from 37 countries on the likelihood of poor COVID-19 outcomes in HIV-positive persons admitted to hospitals for COVID-19 testing. In comparison to those without HIV infection, the chance of developing severe or fatal COVID-19 was 30 per cent higher in PLHIV. Diabetes and hypertension are two frequent underlying diseases in PLHIV. Diabetes and hypertension were linked to an increased risk of death in male PLHIV over the age of 65. These disorders have been linked to an increased risk of serious illness and death [19].

People living with HIV who have co-morbidities (such as chronic lung illness, diabetes, hypertension, obesity, kidney disease, liver disease, Parkinson's disease, multiple sclerosis, and motor neuron disease) should be prioritised for early immunisation and co-morbidity care. Regardless of their immunological status, persons living with HIV should not be omitted from COVID-19 vaccine access plans, and nations should include people living with HIV as a priority group for COVID-19 vaccination based on their epidemiological setting.

As we know that the health care sector got so much burden from the COVID-19 infections but, at the same time nations and WHO collaborates closely to ensure that everyone has fair and equitable access to safe and effective immunizations. Along with the COVID-19 response, it is critical to maintain other critical health services, such as:

- Assisting persons living with HIV to continue taking antiretroviral medication (ART) and adjusting services to make this easier and more efficient throughout the COVID-19 response.
- Maintaining HIV prevention and testing programmes, with a focus on linking to ART introduction.
- Ensuring that patients who begin antiretroviral therapy (ART) can stay on it for the duration of COVID-19 to avoid health risks and problems, including sustaining viral load suppression. This, along with the prevention, diagnosis, and treatment of co-morbidities and co-infections, must be regarded as essential services.
- All persons with HIV and SARS-CoV-2 infections should be monitored, especially those with severe HIV illness or co-morbidities.

VACCINES AGAINST COVID-19

In the United States, where COVID-19 vaccinations are available.

- The US Food and Drug Administration (FDA) has licensed one COVID-19 vaccination and two for emergency use until October 2021.

- Pfizer, Inc. and BioNTech BNT162b2: The FDA approved the Pfizer-BioNTech vaccine, Comirnaty, for people aged 16 and up on August 23, 2021. The vaccination is still available for children and teenagers aged 5 to 15 years old under emergency use authorisation. See what's in the Pfizer COVID-19 vaccine in this infographic.
- ModernaTX, Inc., mRNA-1273: On December 18, 2020, the FDA approved the emergency use of this NIH-funded COVID-19 vaccination for anyone aged 18 and up in the United States. See what's in the Moderna COVID-19 vaccination in this infographic.
- The FDA approved the emergency use of this single-shot vaccine for adults aged 18 and up on February 27, 2021, according to Janssen Pharmaceutical Companies of Johnson & Johnson. This vaccine, which was developed with the help of the National Institutes of Health, does not need to be refrigerated. Women under the age of 50 should be aware of the extremely rare danger of blood clots following vaccination.
- Meanwhile, the Union Health Ministry announced on Tuesday that the total number of COVID-19 vaccine doses delivered in the country had reached 134.53 crores.
- Until 7 p.m., more than 62, 17,862 vaccination doses had been administered. (15th of December, 2021).

Vaccines typically have very high safety requirements and are subject to the most rigorous safety monitoring in the United States.

The timetable for developing the COVID-19 vaccinations was cut in half compared to other vaccines for a variety of reasons:

For decades, scientists at the National Institutes of Health have used and studied mRNA vaccines and coronavirus.

The federal government, scientists, as well as several pharmaceutical businesses teamed up and collaborated like never before, working day and night to share resources and make the operations more effective.

The National Institutes of Health (NIH) established the COVID-19 Prevention Network (COVPN) to coordinate existing research networks and efficiently conduct large clinical studies involving tens of thousands of individuals. Many Americans from all backgrounds volunteered to take part in the study.

The FDA continues to analyse various data and receives immediate updates from clinical trials.

Vaccine Adverse Event Reporting System, called v-safe, is a unique safety system for the authorized COVID-19 vaccines that has been there in existence, where manufacturers of vaccines submit their monthly safety updates to the FDA.

Numerous studies and statistics reveal that immunizations are quite efficient in preventing COVID-19 infection and that being completely vaccinated also helps the individual avoid hospitalisation or death.

Delta Variant

It causes more infections and spreads faster than earlier versions of the virus and may cause more serious illness in unvaccinated individuals.

Vaccines are very successful in the United States, including against the Delta form. Vaccines are highly successful against deadly illnesses, but they aren't flawless, and vaccine-related diseases will occur. As with the surge in cases of the Delta variant, it is expected that thousands of fully vaccinated individuals will become infected and, in turn, infect others. Low vaccination coverage in some parts of the globe will drive the cases further and, in turn, increase the chances of further variants emerging.

Omicron Boosters: Those who are immuno-compromised, such as those on dialysis or immunosuppressants, or who have received an inactivated COVID-19 vaccine - vaccines based on dead SARS CoV 2 - should have booster shots, according to the WHO's Strategic Advisory Group of Experts on Immunization.

The new guidance, according to CDC Director Dr. Rochelle Walensky, indicates the emergence of the omicron variant, and "everyone aged 18 and older should get a booster shot either 6 months after their initial Pfizer or Moderna series or 2 months after their initial J&J vaccine," she said during a statement.

As our body responds to the vaccine uptake, it's normal to have some side effects, which suggests the making of antibodies, and these effects tend to go away in a few days, although not all will have the side effects observed. Serious side effects are, however, unlikely to happen following the vaccination. If a person's health concerns persist after vaccination, it's a good idea to report them to the Vaccine Adverse Event Reporting System (VAERS).

Following mRNA COVID-19 vaccination, certain unusual incidences of cardiac irritation have been documented, mostly in males.

Given the increased risk of serious consequences associated with COVID-19, the CDC continues to recommend vaccination for everyone aged 12 and above.

The National Institutes of Health (NIH) has initiated a clinical trial to evaluate the antibody response to an additional dose of an authorised or licenced COVID-19 vaccination in persons with autoimmune disease who did not respond to the original COVID-19 vaccine regimen. The experiment will also look into whether halting immunosuppressive therapy for autoimmune illness improves antibody response in people who get the second vaccine dose. NIH institutes and centres, in collaboration with private enterprises, continue to explore many types of vaccines in new and current projects.

Current research is attempting to identify whether existing vaccines will provide immunity against evolving COVID-19 variations, or whether new vaccines will be required. Other vaccine studies are continuing to track the health of people who have already received a vaccine to see how effective it is over time.

Often, the clinical trial concept begins in the laboratory. The most promising therapies or procedures are transferred into clinical trials after researchers test them in the lab and on animals. More knowledge about novel medicines, their risks, and their effectiveness is gathered as they progress through a series of processes known as phases.

SUMMARY

- People who had not been fully immunised had a higher chance of testing positive for COVID-19 and dying from COVID-19 than those who had been fully vaccinated.
- In all age categories, unvaccinated people had greater case rates than fully vaccinated people of the same age.
- When compared to individuals in older age groups, those who had been vaccinated between the ages of 12 and 17 had the lowest case rates. Unvaccinated adults aged 50 and up died at higher rates than those in lower age groups, with unvaccinated people aged 80 and up dying at the highest rates.
- Fully vaccinated adults over the age of 80 had a greater death rate than those in lower age groups.
- Because of the low number of deaths from COVID-19 in this age range, death rates among people aged 12-17 are not shown on the graph.

People who were fully vaccinated with any of the three vaccine products (Moderna, Pfizer-BioNTech, Johnson & Johnson's Janssen) had considerably lower case and mortality rates than those who were not.

DATA TABLE

Table 2. Worldwide data of the COVID-19 cases.

Name	Total Number of Cases	Cases Reported in the Last 7 Days	Total Number of Deaths	Deaths in the Last 7 Days that have been Freshly Reported	Total Number of Vaccination Doses given Per 100 People	Per 100 People, the Number of People Who have been Fully Vaccinated
Global By World Bank Income Group High-income Lower Income Lower middle-income Upper middle-income	261,435,768 251,856 543 37,407 105,304	3,882,967 2,694,188 4,928 326,004 843,812	5,207,634 2,192 23 1,203 2,469	48,559 19,234 205 10,137 18,872	99.72 148.916 8.087 65.303 134.911	41.32 64.57 3.17 24.38 57.38
India	34,587,822	61,342	468,980	2,833	85.766	29.92
United Arab Emirates	741,976	476	2,146	2	220.867	-
Qatar	243,290	1,062	611	-	172.558	-
Singapore	263,486	9,837	710	43	159.4	79.236
Cambodia	120,112	208	2,935	30	169.81	79.151
Republic of Korea	447,230	26,281	3,624	296	158.45	78.982
Malaysia	2,627,903	36,417	30,370	307	159.16	77.054
Canada	1,782,171	14,380	29,618	115	158.91	76.509
Ireland	564,657	30,063	5,652	43	160.7	76.164
Denmark	483,253	29,451	2,883	67	152.7	75.962
Japan	1,727,221	699	18,359	10	154.57	75.95
Belgium	1,749,469	94,571	26,966	261	157.5	75.119
Spain	5,153,924	53,971	88,008	90	158.4	74.193
Bhutan	2,640	7	3	-	149.47	73.113
Italy	5,015,790	83,699	133,739	492	155.9	72.929
Finland	186,538	6,702	1,335	4	152.9	72.285
Australia	209,142	9,508	1,997	49	150.71	71.802
Norway	260,920	16,499	1,050	13	149.5	70.796
New Zealand	11,206	1,181	44	4	148.69	70.174
Israel	1,343,075	3,537	8,195	14	146.1	69.593

(Table 2) cont.....

Name	Total Number of Cases	Cases Reported in the Last 7 Days	Total Number of Deaths	Deaths in the Last 7 Days that have been Freshly Reported	Total Number of Vaccination Doses given Per 100 People	Per 100 People, the Number of People Who have been Fully Vaccinated
France	7,394,153	203,051	116,545	461	153	69.362
China	127,814	277	5,697	-	165.37	68.98
Netherlands	2,621,022	155,967	19,349	355	140.4	68.83
Germany	5,836,813	405,902	101,344	1,911	141.4	67.976
The United Kingdom	10,189,063	299,133	144,810	838	165.4	67.835
Sweden	1,198,848	7,243	15,145	1	146.1	67.716
Maldives	91,543	599	250	2	140.17	67.03
Mongolia	381,330	2,936	1,922	37	151.29	65.492
Austria	1,149,939	82,084	11,987	342	145.6	64.501
Saudi Arabia	549,720	202	8,834	8	135.89	64.285
Sri Lanka	563,267	4,407	14,328	146	138.41	64.078
Argentina	5,326,448	11,100	116,529	152	147.05	64.047
Brazil	22,080,906	63,630	614,278	1,619	144.42	63.332
Ecuador	526,615	2,262	33,219	94	139.79	63.277
Switzerland	1,001,561	38,547	11,069	66	128.9	62.458
Morocco	949,785	809	14,775	11	132.16	61.583
Greece	931,183	44,976	18,067	642	129.2	61.466
Turkey	8,770,372	173,962	76,635	1,400	141.5	60.174
United States of America	47,945,945	508,779	773,083	5,787	148.99	59.573
Hungary	1,103,108	70,893	34,521	1,178	136.8	58.879
Thailand	2,115,872	39,737	20,771	282	123.1	56.164
Peru	2,234,075	9,731	201,108	242	122.83	53.787
Poland	3,540,061	162,238	83,583	2,354	101.9	53.509
Iran	6,113,192	30,327	129,711	658	121.27	53.113
Mexico	3,883,842	19,572	293,897	1,373	102.45	50.282
Colombia	5,065,373	17,312	128,437	344	110.45	47.818
Oman	304,519	20	4,113	-	103.24	45.224
Serbia	1,252,573	16,745	11,637	356	91.7	44.697
Kazakhstan	1,054,091	6,596	17,845	143	88.3	42.215

(Table 2) cont.....

Name	Total Number of Cases	Cases Reported in the Last 7 Days	Total Number of Deaths	Deaths in the Last 7 Days that have been Freshly Reported	Total Number of Vaccination Doses given Per 100 People	Per 100 People, the Number of People Who have been Fully Vaccinated
Vietnam	1,224,110	119,275	25,055	1,104	107.62	39.706
North Macedonia	215,125	2,751	7,569	113	77.2	37.903

CONCLUSION

We discovered evidence in our study that supports the idea that COVID-19 has a most common order of recognisable symptoms that is distinct from other prevalent respiratory diseases. In the three diseases studied that are caused by coronaviruses (*i.e.*, COVID-19, SARS, and MERS), fever is the most common initial symptom, followed by cough in influenza. In MERS and SARS, the most likely order of the four recognisable symptoms is the same, but COVID-19's most likely course differs in one important way. Fever and cough are the first two signs of COVID-19, SARS, and MERS. In COVID-19, however, the upper GI tract (nausea/vomiting) appears to be damaged before the lower GI tract (diarrhoea), which is the polar opposite of MERS. We discovered that the beginning symptoms of the most likely path were the same as the most likely path of the four detectable symptoms when we looked at a set of seven symptoms that included three subjective ones (sore throat, headache, and myalgia). In addition, the GI tract symptoms come last in both the four and seven symptom implementations. Fever, myalgia, cough, and diarrhoea were listed as the symptoms with the highest to lowest probability in a distinct MERS dataset, with fever, myalgia, cough, and diarrhoea listed as the symptoms with the highest to lowest probability [20]. This sequence resembles the most plausible path that we discovered. Diarrhoea was the first symptom for only a tiny percentage of patients. As every patient in this dataset who originally experienced diarrhoea subsequently developed pneumonia or respiratory failure, this study demonstrates that diarrhoea as an early symptom indicates more severe disease. These patients may have had a more aggressive form of the disease and have rushed through the most likely path, having already had diarrhoea, according to our hypothesis. These findings are consistent with another dataset provided for SARS, which included the percentage of people who reported the various symptoms first. Fever is the most commonly reported symptom, followed by cough or dyspnea, and finally, diarrhoea, which was reported by a tiny percentage of patients [21]. This sequence reaffirms the most likely direction we've figured out. The fact that diarrhoea was a very uncommon first symptom with a non-zero likelihood of incidence is in line with our findings. This supports our notion that the early onset of diarrhoea indicates a much more aggressive type of disease in those people.

CONSENT FOR PUBLICATION

Not applicable.

CONFLICT OF INTEREST

The authors declare no conflict of interest, financial or otherwise.

ACKNOWLEDGEMENTS

Declared none.

REFERENCES

[1] [1] Ping K, Lei M, Gou Y, Tao Y, Huang Y. Epidemiologic Characteristics of COVID-19 in Guizhou, China. MedRxiv 2013. 2020-03. [http://dx.doi.org/10.1101/2020.03.01.20028944]

[2] Xiang N, Havers F, Chen T, *et al.* Use of national pneumonia surveillance to describe influenza A(H7N9) virus epidemiology, China, 2004-2013. Emerg Infect Dis 2013; 19(11): 1784-90. [http://dx.doi.org/10.3201/eid1911.130865] [PMID: 24206646]

[3] Vong S, O'Leary M, Feng Z. Early response to the emergence of influenza A(H7N9) virus in humans in China: the central role of prompt information sharing and public communication. Bull World Health Organ 2014; 92(4): 303-8. [http://dx.doi.org/10.2471/BLT.13.125989] [PMID: 24700999]

[4] Lotfi M, Hamblin MR, Rezaei N. COVID-19: Transmission, prevention, and potential therapeutic opportunities. Clin Chim Acta 2020; 508: 254-66. [http://dx.doi.org/10.1016/j.cca.2020.05.044] [PMID: 32474009]

[5] Chinazzi M, Davis JT, Ajelli M, *et al.* The effect of travel restrictions on the spread of the 2019 novel coronavirus (COVID-19) outbreak. Science 2020; 368(6489): 395-400. [http://dx.doi.org/10.1126/science.aba9757] [PMID: 32144116]

[6] (WHO) WHO. https://www.who.int/news/item/30-01-2020-statement-on-the-second-meeting-of-the-international-health-regulations-(2005)-emergency-committee-regarding-the-outbreak-of-novel-coronavirus-(2019-ncov)

[7] Sun X, Wandelt S, Zheng C, Zhang A. COVID-19 pandemic and air transportation: Successfully navigating the paper hurricane. J Air Transp Manage 2021; 94102062. [http://dx.doi.org/10.1016/j.jairtraman.2021.102062] [PMID: 33875908]

[8] Kamel Boulos MN, Geraghty EM. Geographical tracking and mapping of coronavirus disease COVID-19/severe acute respiratory syndrome coronavirus 2 (SARS-CoV-2) epidemic and associated events around the world: how 21st century GIS technologies are supporting the global fight against outbreaks and epidemics. Int J Health Geogr 2020; 19(1): 8. [http://dx.doi.org/10.1186/s12942-020-00202-8] [PMID: 32160889]

[9] Kupferschmidt K, Wadman M. Delta variant triggers new phase in the pandemic. Science 2021; 372(6549): 1375-6. [http://dx.doi.org/10.1126/science.372.6549.1375]

[10] Ettaboina SK, Nakkala K, Laddha K. A Mini Review on SARS-COVID-19-2 Omicron Variant (B.

1.1. 529). SciMedicine Journal 2021; 3: 399-406.
[http://dx.doi.org/10.28991/SciMedJ-2021-0304-10]

[11] Do Psychiatry, NIoMHN NIMHANS. Mental Health in the times of COVID-19 Pandemic Guidance for General Medical and Specialised Mental Health Care Settings 2020.

[12] Guo X, Gupta A, Sampat A, Zhai C. A stochastic contact network model for assessing outbreak risk of COVID-19 in workplaces. PLoS One 2022; 17(1): e0262316.
[http://dx.doi.org/10.1371/journal.pone.0262316] [PMID: 35030206]

[13] Larsen JR, Martin MR, Martin JD, Kuhn P, Hicks JB. Modeling the Onset of Symptoms of COVID-19. Front Public Health 2020; 8: 473.
[http://dx.doi.org/10.3389/fpubh.2020.00473] [PMID: 32903584]

[14] Lauer SA, Grantz KH, Bi Q, *et al.* The Incubation Period of Coronavirus Disease 2019 (COVID-19) From Publicly Reported Confirmed Cases: Estimation and Application. Ann Intern Med 2020; 172(9): 577-82.
[http://dx.doi.org/10.7326/M20-0504] [PMID: 32150748]

[15] Koichi Y, Miho F, Sophia K. COVID-19 pathophysiology: A review, Clinical Immunology, Volume 215 2020; 215: 108427.

[16] WHO. WHO SAGE Roadmap For Prioritizing Uses Of COVID-19 Vaccines In The Context Of Limited Supply. https://www.who.int/publications/m/item/who-sage-roadmap-for-prioritizing-u-es-of-cOVID-19-vaccines-in-the-context-of-limited-supply

[17] BHABTHTT. guidance, SARS-CoV-2 vaccine advice for adults living with HIV: British HIV Association (BHIVA) & Terrence Higgins Trust (THT) guidance - Plain English version, 2021.

[18] Bhaskaran K, Rentsch CT, MacKenna B, *et al.* HIV infection and COVID-19 death: a population-based cohort analysis of UK primary care data and linked national death registrations within the OpenSAFELY platform. Lancet HIV 2021; 8(1): e24-32.
[http://dx.doi.org/10.1016/S2352-3018(20)30305-2] [PMID: 33316211]

[19] Bertagnolio S, Thwin S, Silva R. *et al.,* Clinical characteristics and prognostic factors in people living with HIV hospitalized with COVID-19: findings from the WHO Global Clinical Platform. 11th International AIDS Society Conference on HIV Science 2021.

[20] WHO. Organization WH Organization WH. Report of the WHO-China Joint Mission on Coronavirus Disease 2019 (Covid-19). (2020). Available online at: www.who.int/docs/default-source/coronaviruse/who-china-joint-mission-on-covid-19-final-report.pdf

[21] Guan W, Ni Z, Hu Y, *et al.* Clinical Characteristics of Coronavirus Disease 2019 in China. N Engl J Med 2020; 382(18): 1708-20.
[http://dx.doi.org/10.1056/NEJMoa2002032] [PMID: 32109013]

CHAPTER 2

Hypothetical Study on Organophosphates and SARS-CoV-2 Collaborating in Causing Several Respiratory and Immune Diseases for Future Generation: A Review

Nitya Dubey[1,*], Tahmeena Khan[2], Pavan Kumar Nagar[1], Brijesh Singh[1] and **Anju Verma[1]**

[1] *Indian Institute of Technology, Kanpur, Uttar Pradesh, India*

[2] *Department of Chemistry, Integral University, Lucknow, India*

Abstract: Increasing population and increased intensity of crop production led to the invention of pesticides, among which organophosphates are extensively commercialized and used as commercial pesticides. Their toxicity leads to millions of deaths every year. The insecticide enters the food web and inhibits acetyl-cholinesterase enzyme production, which upturns into respiratory dysfunctioning and immuno-toxic production. SARS-CoV-2, a natural micro immuno-toxin, serves a similar mechanism over our body. It affects both the respiratory system and autoimmunity. The scope of this review article is to brief and explain the mechanism and relation between these two co-partners and their futuristic impact on the world. Henceforth, it is also recommended to utilize cost-effective homemade natural pesticides and integrated farming practices to provide secure and healthy food production and curb the future health hazards caused by SARS-CoV-2 and organophosphates.

Keywords: Immune-toxins, Natural Pesticides, Organic Farming, Organophosphates, Pesticides, SARS-CoV-2.

INTRODUCTION

Pesticides, an ingredient that prevents, destroys, repels, or mitigates any pest, are classified as Herbicides, Rodenticides, Fungicides, and Bactericides used to control pest-induced diseases and improve crop yields. These dominant factors are the leading cause of using pesticides. But, after the famous identification of Bernardino Ramazzini that farmers are prone to Ramazzini's syndrome (an acute

* **Corresponding author Nitya Dubey:** Indian Institute of technology-Kanpur, Uttar Pradesh, India;
E-mail: nitya13.1995@gmail.com

pulmonary disease of farmers related to threshing grain), it is comprehensible that pesticides would provide the same results due to their toxic chemical composition [1]. In 1952, India established the production plant for the production and manufacturing of BHC in Calcutta. It was being reported that in 1958, the production rate was 5,000 metric tons, and in 1998, 102, 240 metric tons. As the demand for pesticides increased in 1996-1997, the estimated value reached Rs. 2 billion, *i.e.*, 0.5 billion USD. This was two percent of the total world market. Unfortunately, due to different usage patterns, extensive production and exposure to pesticides have created "a pesticide-based disease havoc" worldwide [2]. Pesticides are also exposed to children through various routes from prenatal to post-development stages that result in severe respiratory illnesses. Many studies [3] have reported that 79% of cases are found to be positively linked to pesticide vulnerabilities and cause respiratory infections (*e.g.*, asthma, coughs, wheezing, acute respiratory diseases, eczema, rhinitis, lung function impairments, and chronic phlegm). An anti-cholinesterase insecticide named organophosphate (OPs) (Fig. **1**) has become a global threat today. The use of diazinon ruins the mechanism of the acetylcholinesterase enzyme in the body and destroys the proper functioning of nerve signaling. It damages the mechanism of the human nervous system and harms the anatomy of tiny organisms like insects, which eventually pass to humans through the food web [4].

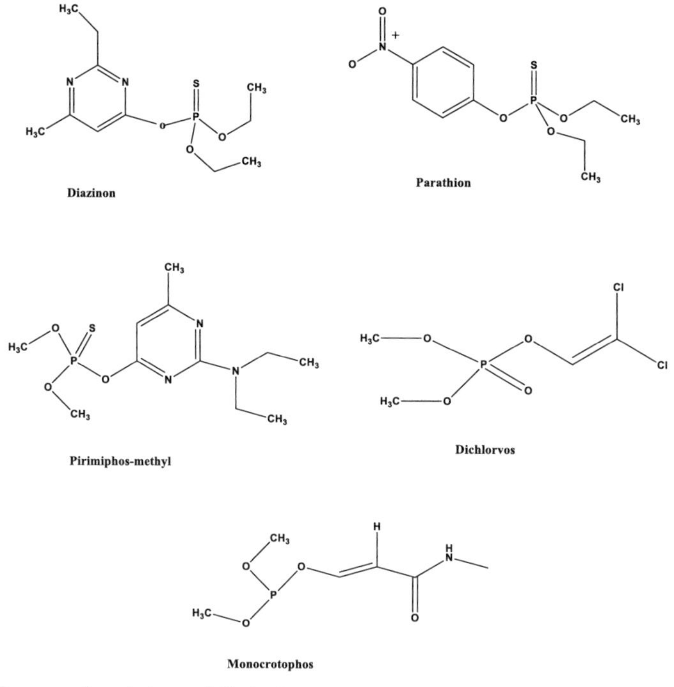

Fig. (1). Types of organophosphates and their structures.

A study conducted in Madhya Pradesh, Bhopal, and Faizabad showed the overuse of pesticides like HCH isomers, Malathion (Table **1**), endosulfan, chlorpyrifos, and methyl-parathion were responsible for degrading the mother's milk which is conceivably harmful to the infants [5, 6]. Consumption of OPs like endosulfan (8.6 times) by newborn babies *via* breast milk and Malathion (4.1) crosses the excessive set consumption limit by World Health Organization in a different area. It implies that the use of endosulfan is more than Malathion, and sincere attention is needed to avoid respiratory infection. The nervous system damaged by endosulfan and other OPs is more inclined to immuno-toxicant spreading among human beings and non-targeted species [5].

Table 1. Examples of pesticides causing acute respiratory infections in humans.

Pesticides	Structure	Toxicity Effect	References
Monocrotophos	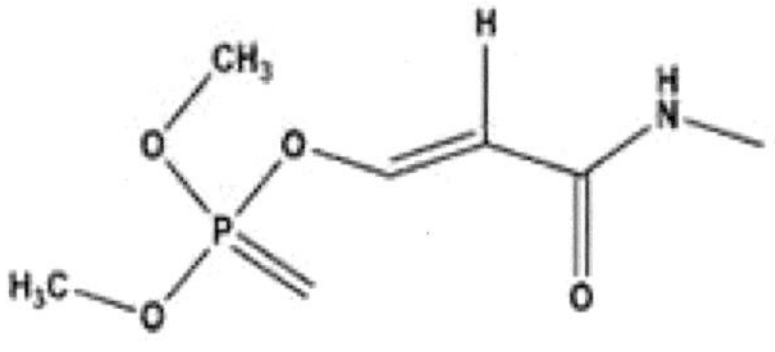 Monocrotophos	Acute exposure responsible for a decrease in the consumption of oxygen.	[7]
Malathion	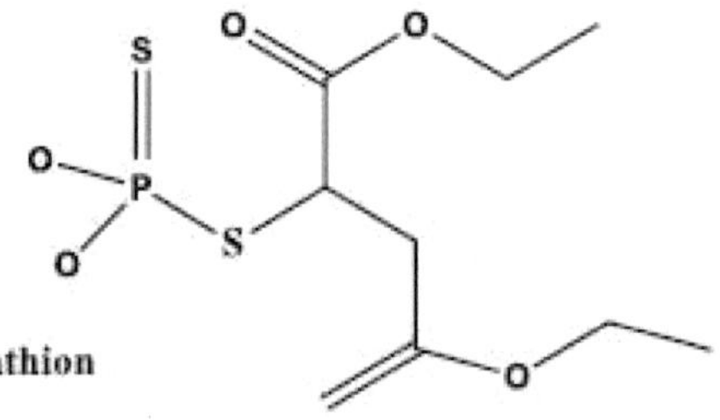 Malathion	Famous for the inhibition of acetylcholinesterase enzyme, damages DNA, destroys the cellular activities responsible for antioxidant defense mechanism and facilitates the destruction of apoptotic cells.	[8]
Coumaphos	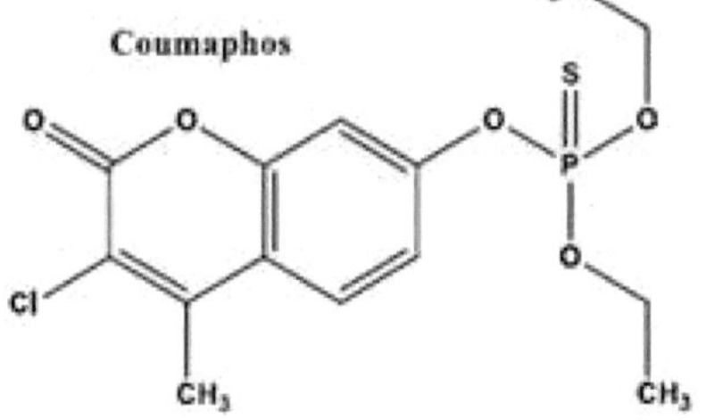 Coumaphos	Allergic asthma was caused by Coumaphos (OR 2.34; 95% CI 1.49–3.70)	[9]

(Table 1) cont.....

Pesticides	Structure	Toxicity Effect	References
Permethrin	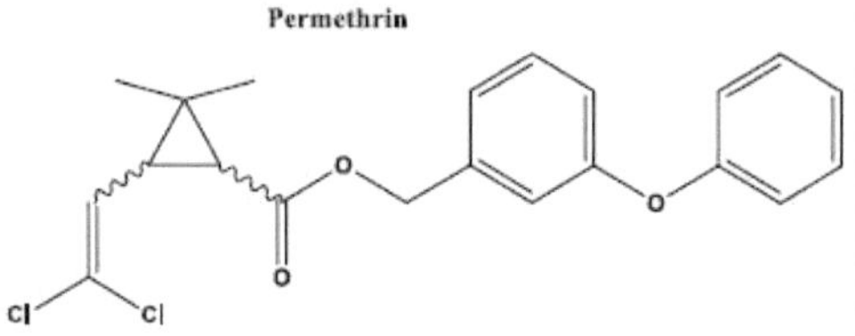	The U.S. Environmental Protection Agency has considered Permethrin a carcinogen due to its tumors production in lungs in female mice and liver tumors in mice of both sexes.	[10]

Respiratory Effects upon Exposure and Usage of Pesticides

Pesticides are largely used for maximum agricultural output and pest control purposes. Initially, organochlorine was considered best in combating several diseases, like typhus and malaria but got prohibited after the 1960s in most countries. Then, organophosphates (the 1960s), Carbamates (1970s), and Pyrethroids (1980s) were the milestones for the agricultural fields. Pesticides toxicity became a worldwide threat when excessively used to produce a maximum yield in a short period of time and become baleful to non-targeted species, including human beings. Cases of Acute respiratory infection and cancer due to pesticide exposure have become prominent in every country [11].

The mechanism of pesticide toxicity in the respiratory system occurs due to exposure to highly volatile pesticide products. Symptom comprises airway irritation, wheezing, sore/dry throat, breathlessness, chest congestion, nose secretion, dyspnea, cough, and lung cancer [12]. A study conducted by a group of researchers in the bottling plant successfully overviews the present and futuristic respiratory risks from pesticide exposure. They have found throat irritation in males (OR = 2.35, 95% CI: 1.10-3.50), nasal dryness (OR= 1.19, 95% CI: 1.10-3.15 in males; OR= 1.15, 95% CI: 1.105-2.91 in females), nasal catarrh (OR= 2.15, 95% CI: 1.15- 4.10 in males; OR = 2.15, 95% CI: 1.12- 3.40 in females), chronic cough in females (OR= 1.29, 95% CI: 1.15- 15.84), nasal dryness (OR = 1.19, 95% CI: 1.10–3.15 in males; OR = 1.15, 95% CI: 1.05–2.91 in females) and dyspnea grades 3 and 4 (OR = 2.35, 95% CI: 1.50–4.10 in males; OR = 1.11, 95% CI: 1.06–1.97 in females) [13]. Hoppin *et al.* had shown in their research that there are eleven pesticides, organophosphates (dichlorvos, parathion, Malathion, diazinon, coumaphos), Organochlorine pesticide (DDT, toxaphene, lindane, and heptachlor chlordane), carbamate pesticide (carbofuran and carbaryl), chlorophenoxy herbicides, Permethrin, petroleum oil, and chlorimuron-ethyl are notably associated with acute respiratory illness such as chronic bronchitis in American Agriculture Health Study (AHS). In another study of AHS, higher exposure to pesticides (OR= 1.85, 95% CI: 1.51-2.25) among farmers results in chronic bronchitis [14].

Asthma exacerbations are generally associated with pesticide exposure. In Australia, a retrospective cohort study of outdoor pesticide applicators was conducted (SMR= 3.45; 95% CI: 1.39-7.10) in which the cases of mortality rate from asthma was high. The workers were exposed to carbaryl, chlorpyrifos, and Organochlorine insecticide DDT [15].

Chemical Reaction and Toxicokinetics of Pesticides

The severity of pesticide toxicity is generally recognized by chemical characterization, dose, route, and duration of exposure [16]. To identify the chemical aspects of the toxicology of pesticides, a better understanding of Toxicodynamic and Toxicokinetics interactions is required. Different pesticides, when they come in contact with the human body then, alter the predicted metabolic pathways.

Toxicokinetics interaction occurs due to the effect of one pesticide on the other pesticides by altering their absorption, distribution, elimination, or metabolism methods. It occurs at all doses level, but the effect has not been seen at low doses [17]. The most prominent effect of such interactions accompanies the change in the relationship between the external dose and the analogous level of a pesticide at its target site. Toxicodynamic interactions need an adequate amount of pesticide to reach the target tissue and source out a disturbance in physiology. The second toxicant is responsible for the same perturbation, which further exacerbates or antagonizes the first compound. The main necessity for the toxicodynamic interactions is a sufficient amount of pesticide that surpasses the threshold effect [18].

The combination of toxicological effects of more than two pesticides can be explained in three forms, which are independent, dose addition, or interaction. An independent interaction occurs when the individual pesticides have a different mode of action or mechanism than the mixture of pesticides to which it is added. The conclusion of such interaction shows a peculiar default assumption of the combined exposure of the effect of the mixture of pesticides results in toxicity when the threshold effect of the pesticide is high in the consumer [19].

Dose addition is taken in the case of mixtures of pesticides that produce a similar toxic effect by influencing the same target organ through the same toxicity mechanism over the whole dose range [20]. When two pesticides follow the same toxicity mechanism or biochemical mechanism and target the same tissue, they viably share a common toxic intermediate [21]. The additive effect results from the chemical interactions (Fig. **2**). These interactions show a deviation from simple additivity due to individual components or compounds out-turns the toxicity of one another [22]. Therefore, the combined effect of more than two pesticides is greater (Synergistic, supra-additive, potentiating) or less (antagonistic, infra-additive, inhibitive) in comparison to the predicted on the basis of response addition or dose addition [19].

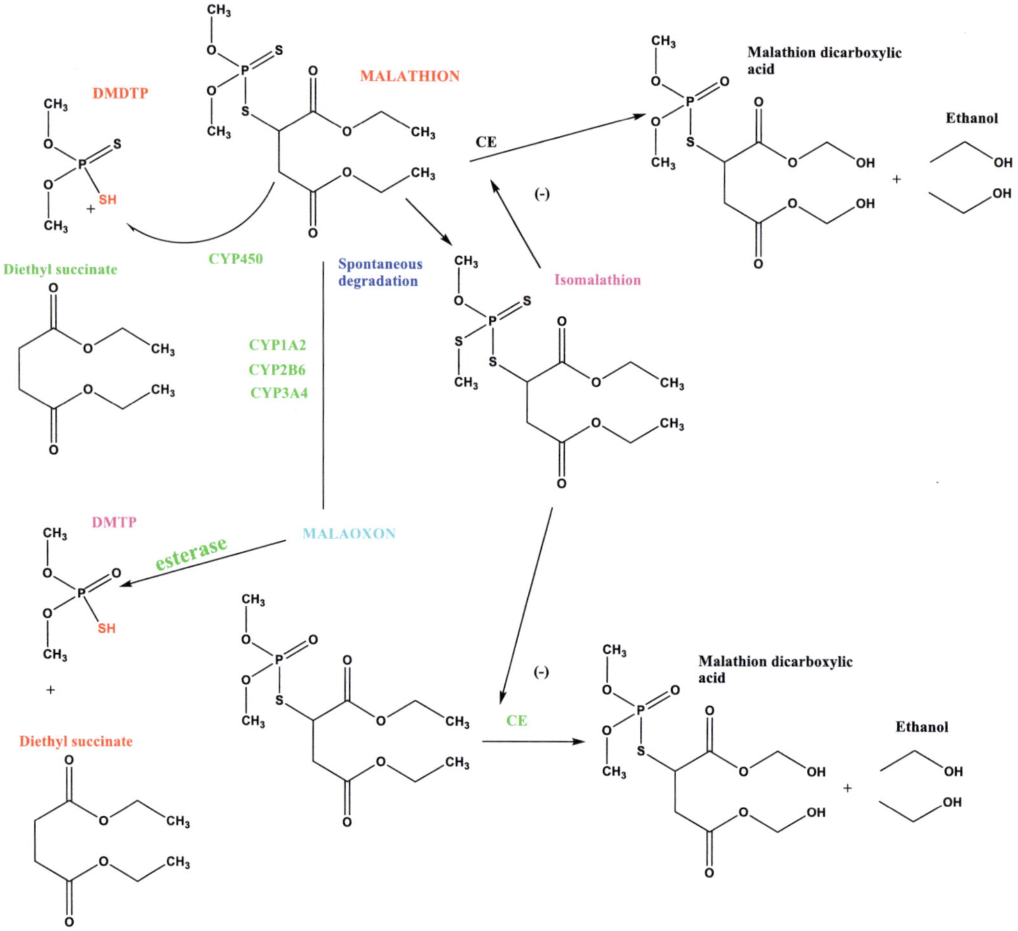

Fig. (2). Potentiation of Malathion toxicity by isolation [16].

On Dec 31, 2019, the first outbreak of COVID-19 was reported in Wuhan, China, drawn out by the SARS-CoV-2 (Severe Acute Respiratory Syndrome Coronavirus-2). Then, WHO (World Health Organization) in July 2020 announced it was the newest pandemic in the world. Coronavirus or novel coronavirus-infected pneumonia (NCIP) is a contagious disease spread through sneezing, speaking or coughing micro-droplets aerosol from the infected person. It is also spread by touching contaminated utensils, clothes, furniture, and related surfaces.

Research conducted by Baig *et al.* [23] reported that the SARS-CoV-2 seed's alveolar vandalization consolidates lung parenchyma and pneumonia in the human body and sets off the alteration in gases dispensed in the blood of the infected person that gives rise to severe issues like a hypoxemic respiratory failure. However, if we compare the facts, then exposure to pesticides is accountable for oxidative stress in the body, which in due course is accountable for causing respiratory dysfunction and detainment of the immune health. Unfortunately, Covid-19 and SARS-CoV-2 share a similar destruction process in damaging the functioning of the respiratory system and disarming the proper function of the immune system. However, it means that pesticides like organophosphate and SARS-CoV-2 serve the same dish, *i.e.*, respiratory failure and immunity deterioration, but through different mechanisms. This review chapter will discuss the comparative study between pesticides and SARS-CoV-2, sharing a similar conviction to vandalize the immune and respiratory systems in humans.

ORGANOPHOSPHATES AND SARS-COV-2: MECHANISM TO DAMPEN THE FUNCTIONING OF RESPIRATORY AND IMMUNE SYSTEM

The first organophosphate was reported in the mid-1800s but not utilized in the period of World War II. Its main merits conclude that it is helpful in the field of medication, and pest management. Severe exposure to OPs includes tear and saliva production, diarrhea, vomiting, small pupils, muscle tremors, sweating, confusion and diarrhea. The molecule of OPs can be absorbed through the skin, inhalation, or the presence of its content in the gastrointestinal tract (Fig. **3**). The absorption results in linkage with acetylcholinesterase molecule in RBCs, thus making the enzyme non-functional or inactive. Mechanism future follows on the neuromuscular junctions, in which the overstimulation of nicotinic receptors leads to myoclonic and fasciculation jerks that result in flaccid paralysis due to depolarizing block [24 - 27]. Organophosphate pesticides inhibit carboxyl ester hydrolase production, which mainly results in acetylcholinesterase (AChE) inhibition. It inactivates the AChE by phosphorylation of the serine hydroxyl group, followed by an assemblage of acetylcholine which overstimulates the muscarinic receptors.

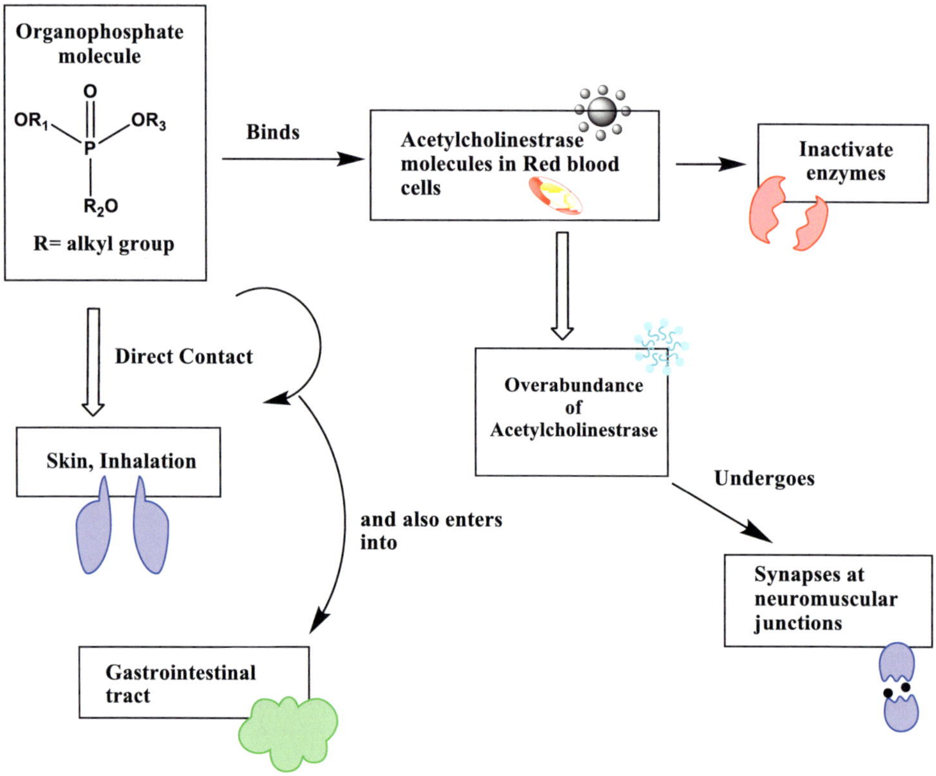

Fig. (3). Toxicokinesis: On exposure to organophosphates.

SARS-COV-2

Coronavirus Disease (COVID-19) elicited by Sever Acute Respiratory Syndrome Coronavirus 2 (SARS-CoV-2) comes under the group of beta-coronavirus. It is a single and positive-stranded ribonucleic acid virus, which is responsible for SARS-CoV-2 in humans [28].

Morphology

It possesses four structural proteins that are nucleocapsid protein (N), E (envelope), and M (membrane). Nucleocapsid proteins assist in the formation of a helical capsid for the accommodation of the virus genome. Then lipid membrane surrounds the whole structure, which is made up of S (spike), E (envelope) and M (membrane) proteins. Spike proteins are required for the virus entry and recognition of the host cells. S protein helps in the formation of large protrusions, also known as Peplomers, on the virus's surface. Peplomers provide crown-like shape or "CORONA" like shape (the term corona is derived from the Latin word crown). Corona comprises three segments: the large ectodomain, the transmembrane domain and the intracellular tail. The subunits S1 and S2 (receptor binders) are positioned in the ectodomain region, which plays a significant role during infection. The host receptors are wrapped with S1, and S2 merges the host and viral membranes to release the virus's genome into the host cell [29].

Biochemistry

The genome of SARS-CoV-2 consists of 30,000 nucleotides that encode four structural proteins, *i.e.*, Spike (S protein), Envelope (E) protein, Membrane (M) protein and Nucleocapsid (N) protein. During infection, the most abundantly expressed protein is the N protein which is very immunogenic. N-proteins enter together with the viral RNA into the host body after infection. It can also bind with a non-specific dsDNA due to its electrostatic interaction. It contains two distinct RNA- binding domains, C- terminal domain (CTD] and N- terminal domain [NTD], which are linked with a poor structure linkage region (LKR). LKR contains an arginine-rich/ serine (SR-rich) domain (SRD). The viral RNA genome binds with the positive amino acid, SARS-CoV N- CTD and N-NTD [30].

In searching the quick treatment for COVID-19, it was found that the serological diagnosis detects the specific antibodies against the N-protein in the patients of SARS. It shows high sensitivity and persistence in comparison to the other structural proteins of SARS-CoV-2. It is also detected that the anti-N antibodies have been seen in the early stage of infection. The positive results shown by the N-proteins will increase the chances and our understanding towards COVID-19 which will help us to frame better biological designs to identify and cure the patients suffering from it [30].

Physiology and Mechanism

The virus entry follows two steps: The first is the endocytic pathway, and the second is the non-endosomal pathway [31] (Fig. **4**).The most extensively used pathway for studying SARS-CoV-2 and MERS-CoV viral entry is the endocytic pathway. SARS-CoV-2 uses the same receptors; hence, Wang *et al.* [32] reported that the SARS-CoV-2 uses clathrin- and caveolae-independent endocytic pathways for viral entry.

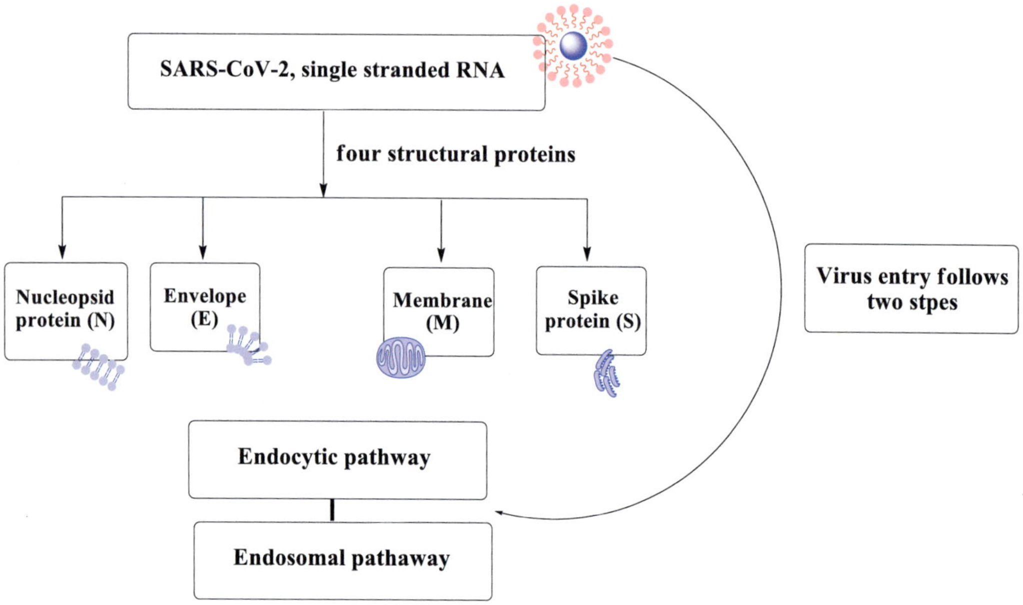

Fig. (4). SARS-CoV-2: Structural proteins and entry pathways.

During viral infection, spike proteins (~ 1300 amino acid residues) are divided by host proteases in the receptor-binding subunit called S1, then into the membrane fusion subunit S2. The S1 subunit wraps up with the sugar receptors and ACE2 during cell entry. S2 protein then goes through conformational changes and attains a post-fusion state (Fig. **5**). This state includes the three pairs of the heptad region HR-N and HR-C. HR-C and HR-N in the form of the trimeric S2, a six-helix bundle structure [33]. These transmembrane anchors and fusion peptides are oriented at the end of the six-helix bundle structure, bringing the host and viral membranes to fusion [34]. This process releases a large amount of energy which accelerates and forwards the membrane fusion [29]. Spike proteins have a high binding affinity with the sugar receptors of human cells, indicating that SARS-CoV-2 (spike proteins) has an association with the sugar receptors of human cells and ACE2. The spike proteins of SARS-CoV-2 bind with the peptidase domain (PD) of ACE2 with a K_d (equilibrium dissociation constant) of ~ 15 Nm [35]. SARS-CoV-2 enters the host cells through endocytosis, and cathepsin L and cathepsin B lysosomal proteases process its spike protein. The elastase, an extracellular protease in the respiratory tract, and TMPRSS2 (transmembrane proteases essential for smooth entry of the virus) [36] present on the surface of lung cells activate the spike membrane fusion.

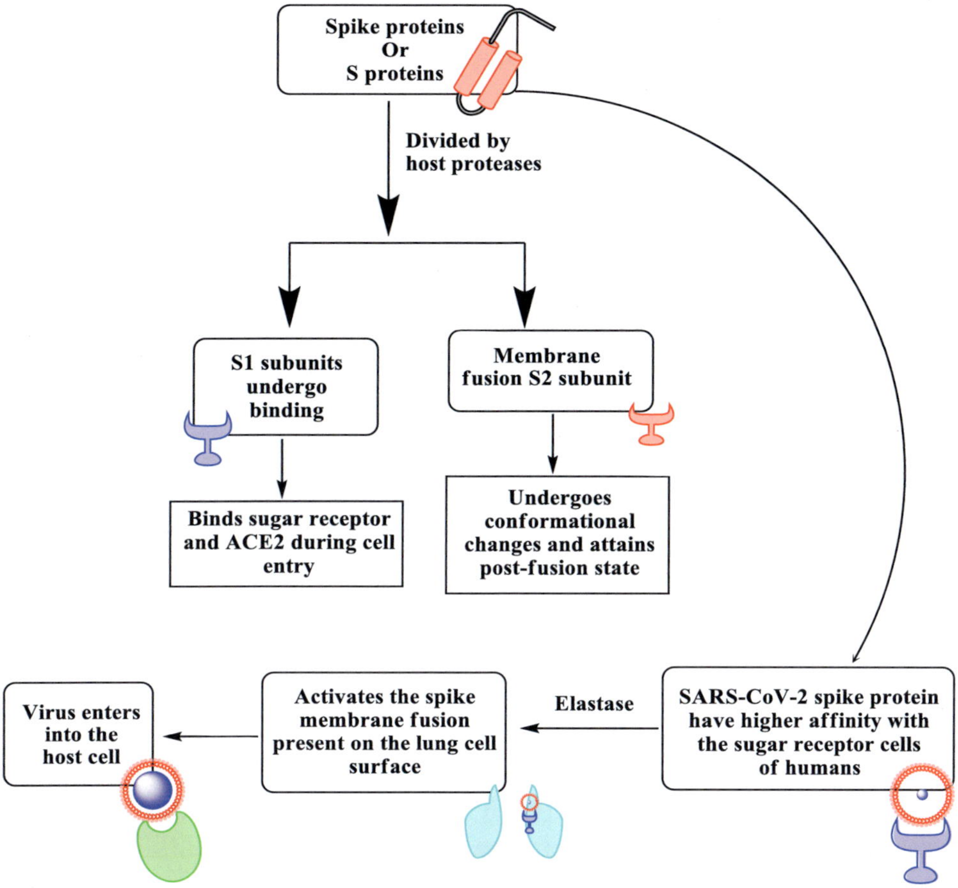

Fig. (5). SARS-CoV-2: Mechanism of attack on the host cells.

This process releases a large amount of energy which accelerates and forwards the membrane fusion [29]. Spike proteins have a high binding affinity with the sugar receptors of human cells, indicating that the SARS-CoV-2 (spike proteins) has an affinity with the sugar receptors of human cells and ACE2. The spike proteins of SARS-CoV-2 bind with the peptidase domain (PD) of ACE2 with a K_d (equilibrium dissociation constant) of ~ 15 Nm [35]. Through endocytosis, SARS-CoV-2 get enters the host cells, and cathepsin L and cathepsin B lysosomal proteases process its spike protein. The elastase, an extracellular protease in the respiratory tract, and TMPRSS2 (transmembrane proteases essential for smooth entry of the virus) [36] present on the surface of lung cells activate the spike membrane fusion.

COMPARATIVE STUDY OF THE IMMUNOTOXICITY MECHANISM AND RESPIRATORY DSYFUNTIONING BETWEEN ORGANO-PHOSPHATE BETWEEN ORGANOPHOSPHATE AND SARS-COV-2

Immunocytes govern the orchestrate cell-mediated response and humoral immune response, which benefits in safeguarding against pathogens like SARS-CoV-2, but when immunocytes are exposed to organophosphate, it alters the working efficiency. It is observed that continuous exposure to the Malathion changes macrophage functioning and mast cell degranulation in mice [37, 38]. Sharing similar examples like the declination caused by dimethyl 2, 2-dichlorovinyl phosphate results in decreased activity of (LAK) lymphokine-activated killer cells, (NK) natural killer, in the cellular system and CTL in a dose-dependent manner [39].

Our immune system plays a crucial role in protecting the body from foreign agents like SARS-CoV-2. The immune response is differentiated into two types, *i.e.*, *innate immune* and *adaptive immune response.* The innate immune response governs the first response against any foreign agent. It is observed that the number of immunocytes count of myeloid lineage is uplifted during this pandemic era in humans. A study conducted on 61 COVID-19 patients showed a high number of neutrophils to lymphocyte ratio and blood neutrophils count [40]. A high count of activated mast cells along with neutrophils has been found in COVID-19 patients in their Bronchoalveolar lavage fluid (BALF) [41, 42]. The initiation of the mechanism of the virus starts from the synthesis of the proinflammatory cytokines like IL-1β,IL-2,IL-6,IL-7,G-CSF,IP-10,MCP-1,MIP-1, TNFα andIL1RA to apply the pyroptosis and cytokine storm in the body [41]. This results in immuno-pathologies developed by the innate defense in the infected patients [43, 44]. There are many other studies [41] that make clear that the complement system and the myeloid cells play a significant role in protecting our immune system, and if the mechanism gets disturbed by any other means, then it will trigger the harmful impact of the virus on the body like bronchitis, respiratory diseases, pneumonia, and acute respiratory distress syndrome (ARDS). Therefore, the innate immune system plays an important role in safeguarding from diseases, mainly in the case of respiratory infections [41].

The *adaptive immune response* includes washing the infected cells created by pathogens facilitated by T- lymphocytes. Nucleocapsid protein-specific antibodies are involved in the humoral immune response [41, 45]. Nucleocapsid proteins specific antibodies and spike RBD-specific *IgM* and *IgGI* antibodies have been detected in the newly cured patients of SARS-CoV-2 infected person [46]. Henceforth, the above few examples proved that somehow both SARS-CoV-2 and OPs obey the exact mechanism in harming the immune system but in their specific ways. The main difference between OPs and SARS-CoV-2 is that organophosphate produces immuno-toxicants, whereas SARS-CoV-2 itself behaves like a micro immuno-toxicant in opposition to the immune system of the body. SARS-CoV-2 directly utilizes ACE-2 receptors to overthrow target cells. SARS-CoV-2 has many structural and non-structural accessory proteins that help in immune function. During infection, it destabilizes the IFN-I [41, 47]; such responses are produced when the STING-TRAF3-TBKI (a type of IFN gene) complex gets agitated by the virus [41, 48]. Also, other proteins of SARS-CoV-2, like NSP15, NSP14, NSP13 and ORF6, turn away the IFN functioning by annihilating the nuclear localization of IRF3 [49]. It is also observed in the early stages of COVID-19 infection that C-reactive proteins can act as an immunosuppressive and obstruct the functioning, activation, and proliferation of $CD8^+$ T-cells and $CD4^+$ [41, 50]. The initiation of infection in the respiratory system starts in the upper airway epitheliums, which eventually harms the alveolar epithelium and disables gaseous exchange functioning. The airway epithelium is regarded as an entry point for the beta-coronavirus, for instance, SARS-CoV-2, MERS-CoV-2, and SARS-CoV. Then, the interaction of Angiotensin-converting enzyme-2 (ACE-2) with the viral proteins accelerates the internalization of the virus into the endosomes. The virus gets to enter the host cell through trans-membrane serine protease-2 (TMPRSS2). The TMPRSS2, for instance, furin breaks down into the S protein to form a fusion protein that acts as a key and helps the virus set foot in the host body [51, 52].

Organophosphate clogs the enzyme AchE that hydrolyzes the neurotransmitter, Ach. Neurotransmitter Ach is located in the cholinergic brain synapses and neuromuscular junction that is governed by Ach receptors within the neuromuscular junctions, central parasympathetic and sympathetic nervous system. Ach receptors employ their activity by using muscarinic or nicotinic cholinergic receptors. Cholinergic transmission is beneficial for respiratory control. Exposures to organophosphates result in phosphorylation of the serine hydroxyl residue on the AchE, inhibiting the assemblage of Ach [53]. Acute exposure to OPs results in a high level of Ach production at the post-junctional with outcomes in abnormal respiratory functioning and central symptoms like delirium, seizures, and central respiratory depression. In contrast, peripheral symptoms include hypotension, paralysis, hypertension, weakness, salivation, diarrhea, mydriasis, muscarinic effects of nausea, urinary incontinency, and bronchorrea. Due to organophosphate exposure, these symptoms are not entirely proven and understood, but it is speculatively assumed that it can disrupt the neuro and respiratory systems [54].

So, consequently, from the above-stated mechanism and examples, we can conclude that Organophosphates and SARS-CoV-2 share a similar infection mechanism; both dampen the autoimmunity and functioning of the respiratory system. Thereupon, by now, it is evident that co-exposure of both the delegates shares a deadly combination to uplift the adversity of the ongoing SARS-CoV-2 pandemic situation or maybe in the future other examples of pesticides offers the exact infecting mechanism with other disease-causing micro-organisms. So, it is recommended to follow the natural methods for farming and getting the better yield.

ALTERNATIVE MEASURES TO GET THE BETTER YIELD WITHOUT USING ORGANOPHOSPHATE PESTICIDES TO SHUN THE FUTURISTIC VULNERABILITY TOWARDS SARS-COV-2

The main aspect of choosing pesticides over natural methods is to curb, feed, better yield, and supply a large crop production to the agricultural world. Still, due to the poisonous nature of pesticides, it has become a major health concern to the world. There are many alternative methods to get better yields without using pesticides, especially in the case of organophosphates. During the 1940s, pesticides weren't invented, yet people practiced farming and obtained desirable productivity from their agricultural fields [55]. Cultural practices include different types of gardening techniques that promote speedy plant growth and impede pests. A Pest-resistant garden plant provides equal benefits to farms, and habitat for wildlife is also applicable the same. Apart from this, plantation of different species, crop rotation, companion-planting, such as marigolds, a natural pest deterrent; management of soil fertility, watering, and proper drainage system to serve a positive optimal growing environment are the other options that can be used relatively instead of pesticides. Biological Control is another alternative that acts upon the same, creating barriers to inhibit snails and slugs using crushed eggshells, oyster shells, and prickly material. The weed growth can be dwindled by mulching between plants, using cloth covers, pouring boiling water on the large weeds like thistles and preventing mildew on sensitive plants. Natural pest control products like natural homemade fungicides prevent blight on tomatoes, black spots on roses, mildew and rust on plants are some natural methods to dampen pest growth [56].

Integrated Farming System or organic farming also serves as a potential method and wise substitution to refine healthy food production. It works on specific protocols conducted, practiced and supervised to protect the integrity of the environment and biodiversity. It supplies higher antioxidants, minerals, and nutrients that enhance immunity and give the body healthy structuring. OPs and SARS CoV-2 release oxidative stress and are highly recommendable to consume antioxidant food to curb the problem [57]. Antioxidant or Immuno protectors can act against immuno-toxicants of OPs like the toxicity of Malathion in the peripheral blood mononuclear cells (PBMC) can be rectified through the curcumin effect and N-acetylcysteine (NAC) [58]. Walnut polyphenols, vitamin E [59], ascorbic acid, zinc oxide nanoparticles [60] and ascorbic acids can act against immuno-toxicants of organophosphates. Antioxidants also stop the process of oxidation and other reactions that are facilitated by free radicals and peroxides. The goods include vitamins E and C, carotenes, essential and non-essential enzymes, and polyphenols. Many researchers have been made to test the food quality to ensure nutritional contents produced by the integrated farming system, *i.e.*, organic farming. Wang *et al.*, 2009 found that the antioxidant content in the case of apples was high when cultivated under organic farming practices [61]. Stracke *et al.* conducted three years comparative study between conventional and organic farming techniques on apples. They found that 15% antioxidant content was reported when the apples were cultivated under organic practices, which was more than in the case of apples grown by conventional methods [62]. Aldrich *et al.*, by following organic farming methods, the content of antioxidants was found to be a high activity, *i.e.* ($P < 0.0001$) ABTS (average of 1546 *vs.* 1387 μmol TEAC kg-1 FWL). DPPH (average of 2194 *vs.* 0.185g kg-1 FW) in tomatoes than grown by conventional methods.

Nowadays, increased food-related awareness in both urban and rural areas results in drastic changes towards healthy lifestyles of people at their own expense. Governments of different countries are paying attention to the promotion of natural and organic farming practices. Henceforth, it is proven and explained that organic farming can produce non-synthetic pesticide food in less time. As we all realize, cultural and biological farming practices will take time, but the result and health concerns are equally important. The above-suggested recommendations are cost-effective and beneficial for both land and the health of wildlife and humans. So, it is highly advisable to draw unfeigned attentiveness towards the topic.

CONCLUSION

The above review shares some noteworthy points regarding the health deterioration of the people. Organophosphate pesticides and SARS-CoV-2 have an indirect friendship in terms of influencing the immune and respiratory systems of the body. They cause pneumonia, asthma, chronic bronchitis and other respiratory infections. As immunotoxins, they might increase the process of pyroptosis, inflammatory reaction and oxidative stress. Today, in this pandemic era, we all know the severity of the situation and not only OPs; many other particles in the environment discombobulate the healthy mechanism of respiratory and immune systems. However, in terms of pesticide toxicity, natural homemade pesticides and organic farming are potential alternatives to obtain healthy and safe food production for future generations. This theoretical study put forward the fundamental idea of the correspondence between the ill health effects caused by SARS-CoV-2 and organophosphates and their alleviation by using natural and cost-effective methods to obtain sustainable development.

CONSENT FOR PUBLICATION

Not applicable.

CONFLICT OF INTEREST

The authors declare no conflict of interest, financial or otherwise.

ACKNOWLEDGEMENTS

The authors are thankful to Prof. Mukesh Sharma, Civil Engineering Department, Indian Institute of Technology Kanpur, for the support.

REFERENCES

[1] Hoppin JA, Umbach DM, London SJ, Lynch CF, Alavanja MCR, Sandler DP. Pesticides and adult respiratory outcomes in the agricultural health study. Ann N Y Acad Sci 2006; 1076(1): 343-54. [http://dx.doi.org/10.1196/annals.1371.044] [PMID: 17119214]

[2] Mathur SC. Future of Indian pesticides industry in next millennium. Pesticide Information 1999; 24(4): 9-23.

[3] Buralli RJ, Dultra AF, Ribeiro H. Respiratory and allergic effects in children exposed to Pesticides—A systematic review. Int J Environ Res Public Health 2020; 17(8): 2740. [http://dx.doi.org/10.3390/ijerph17082740] [PMID: 32316194]

[4] Marrs Timothy C. Organophosphates: history, chemistry, pharmacology. Organophosphates and health 2001; 1-36. [http://dx.doi.org/10.1142/9781848161443_0001]

[5] Sanghi R, Pillai MK, Jayalekshmi TR, Nair A. Organochlorine and organophosphorus pesticide residues in breast milk from Bhopal, Madhya Pradesh, India. Hum Exp Toxicol 2003; 22(2): 73-6. [http://dx.doi.org/10.1191/0960327103ht321oa] [PMID: 12693830]

[6] Srivastava S, Narvi SS, Prasad SC. Levels of select organophosphates in human colostrum and mature milk samples in rural region of Faizabad district, Uttar Pradesh, India. Hum Exp Toxicol 2011; 30(10): 1458-63. [http://dx.doi.org/10.1177/0960327110396525] [PMID: 21247996]

[7] Maniyar RA, Nazeer Ahmed R, David M. Monocrotophos: toxicity evaluation and respiratory responses of *Cyprinus carpio* (Linnaeus). Recent Res Sci Technol 2011; 3(1): 51-4.

[8] Badr AM. Organophosphate toxicity: updates of malathion potential toxic effects in mammals and potential treatments. Environ Sci Pollut Res Int 2020; 27(21): 26036-57. [http://dx.doi.org/10.1007/s11356-020-08937-4] [PMID: 32399888]

[9] Hoppin Jane A, Umbach David M, London Stephanie J, *et al.* Pesticide use and adult-onset asthma among male farmers in the Agricultural Health Study. Eur Respir J 2009; 34: 61296-1303.

[10] Cox C. Permethrin. Global Pesticide Campaigner 1999; 9(3): 20.

[11] Aktar W, Sengupta D, Chowdhury A. Impact of pesticides use in agriculture: their benefits and hazards. Interdiscip Toxicol 2009; 2(1): 1-12.
[http://dx.doi.org/10.2478/v10102-009-0001-7] [PMID: 21217838]

[12] Tarmure S, Alexescu T, Orasan O, *et al.* Influence of pesticides on respiratory pathology – a literature review. Ann Agric Environ Med 2020; 27(2): 194-200.
[http://dx.doi.org/10.26444/aaem/121899] [PMID: 32588592]

[13] Zuskin E, Mustajbegovic J, Schachter EN, *et al.* Respiratory function in pesticide workers. J Occup Environ Med 2008; 50(11): 1299-305.
[http://dx.doi.org/10.1097/JOM.0b013e3181845f6c] [PMID: 19001956]

[14] Hoppin JA, Valcin M, Henneberger PK, *et al.* Pesticide use and chronic bronchitis among farmers in the agricultural health study. Am J Ind Med 2007; 50(12): 969-79.
[http://dx.doi.org/10.1002/ajim.20523] [PMID: 17975796]

[15] Beard J, Sladden T, Morgan G, Berry G, Brooks L, McMichael A. Health impacts of pesticide exposure in a cohort of outdoor workers. Environ Health Perspect 2003; 111(5): 724-30.
[http://dx.doi.org/10.1289/ehp.5885] [PMID: 12727601]

[16] Hernández AF, Parrón T, Tsatsakis AM, Requena M, Alarcón R, López-Guarnido O. Toxic effects of pesticide mixtures at a molecular level: Their relevance to human health. Toxicology 2013; 307: 136-45.
[http://dx.doi.org/10.1016/j.tox.2012.06.009] [PMID: 22728724]

[17] Reffstrup TK, Larsen JC, Meyer O. Risk assessment of mixtures of pesticides. Current approaches and future strategies. Regul Toxicol Pharmacol 2010; 56(2): 174-92.
[http://dx.doi.org/10.1016/j.yrtph.2009.09.013] [PMID: 19782118]

[18] The intergovernmental group on health risks from chemicals. Chemical mixtures: a framework for assessing risk to human health (CR14) Institute of Environment and Health, Cranfield University, Cranfield, UK, 2009. http://ieh.cranfield.ac.uk/ighrc/Chemical%20Mixture%20Final%20May%202009.pdf

[19] Boobis AR, Ossendorp BC, Banasiak U, Hamey PY, Sebestyen I, Moretto A. Cumulative risk assessment of pesticide residues in food. Toxicol Lett 2008; 180(2): 137-50.
[http://dx.doi.org/10.1016/j.toxlet.2008.06.004] [PMID: 18585444]

[20] IGHRC The intergovernmental group on health risks from chemicals Chemical mixtures: a framework for assessing risk to human health (CR14). Cranfield, UK: Institute of Environment and Health, Cranfield University 2009.

[21] U.S. Environmental Protection Agency Policy on a common mechanism of action the organophosphate pesticides Fed Register 1999; 64: 5795-9.

[22] Rider CV, LeBlanc GA. An integrated addition and interaction model for assessing toxicity of chemical mixtures. Toxicol Sci 2005; 87(2): 520-8.
[http://dx.doi.org/10.1093/toxsci/kfi247] [PMID: 16002478]

[23] Baig AM. Computing the Effects of SARS-CoV-2 on Respiration Regulatory Mechanisms in COVID-19. ACS Chem Neurosci 2020; 11(16): 2416-21.
[http://dx.doi.org/10.1021/acschemneuro.0c00349] [PMID: 32600045]

[24] Sikary AK. Homicidal poisoning in India: A short review. J Forensic Leg Med 2019; 61: 13-6.
[http://dx.doi.org/10.1016/j.jflm.2018.10.003] [PMID: 30390552]

[25] Dardiotis E, Aloizou AM, Siokas V, *et al.* Paraoxonase-1 genetic polymorphisms in organophosphate metabolism. Toxicology 2019; 411: 24-31.
[http://dx.doi.org/10.1016/j.tox.2018.10.012] [PMID: 30359673]

[26] Jokanović M. Neurotoxic effects of organophosphorus pesticides and possible association with neurodegenerative diseases in man: A review. Toxicology 2018; 410: 125-31.

[http://dx.doi.org/10.1016/j.tox.2018.09.009] [PMID: 30266654]

[27] Naughton SX, Terry AV Jr. Neurotoxicity in acute and repeated organophosphate exposure. Toxicology 2018; 408: 101-12.
[http://dx.doi.org/10.1016/j.tox.2018.08.011] [PMID: 30144465]

[28] Holmes KV. SARS coronavirus: a new challenge for prevention and therapy. J Clin Invest 2003; 111(11): 1605-9.
[http://dx.doi.org/10.1172/JCI18819] [PMID: 12782660]

[29] Li F. Structure, function, and evolution of coronavirus spike proteins. Annu Rev Virol 2016; 3(1): 237-61.
[http://dx.doi.org/10.1146/annurev-virology-110615-042301] [PMID: 27578435]

[30] Zeng W, Liu G, Ma H, *et al.* Biochemical characterization of SARS-CoV-2 nucleocapsid protein. Biochem Biophys Res Commun 2020; 527(3): 618-23.
[http://dx.doi.org/10.1016/j.bbrc.2020.04.136] [PMID: 32416961]

[31] Zumla A, Chan JFW, Azhar EI, Hui DSC, Yuen KY. Coronaviruses — drug discovery and therapeutic options. Nat Rev Drug Discov 2016; 15(5): 327-47.
[http://dx.doi.org/10.1038/nrd.2015.37] [PMID: 26868298]

[32] Wang H, Yang P, Liu K, *et al.* SARS coronavirus entry into host cells through a novel clathrin- and caveolae-independent endocytic pathway. Cell Res 2008; 18(2): 290-301.
[http://dx.doi.org/10.1038/cr.2008.15] [PMID: 18227861]

[33] Hofmann H, Pöhlmann S. Cellular entry of the SARS coronavirus. Trends Microbiol 2004; 12(10): 466-72.
[http://dx.doi.org/10.1016/j.tim.2004.08.008] [PMID: 15381196]

[34] Shang , Wan , Luo . Cell entry mechanisms of SARS-CoV-2 Proc Natl Acad Sci U S A 2020; 117(21): 11727-34.
[http://dx.doi.org/10.1073/pnas.2003138117]

[35] Wrapp D, Wang N, Corbett KS, *et al.* Cryo-EM structure of the 2019-nCoV spike in the prefusion conformation. Science 2020; 367(6483): 1260-3.
[http://dx.doi.org/10.1126/science.abb2507] [PMID: 32075877]

[36] Gralinski LE, Menachery VD. Return of the Coronavirus: 2019-nCoV. Viruses 2020; 12(2): 135.
[http://dx.doi.org/10.3390/v12020135] [PMID: 31991541]

[37] Rodgers K, Xiong S. Effect of administration of malathion for 14 days on macrophage function and mast cell degranulation. Fundam Appl Toxicol 1997; 37(1): 95-9.
[http://dx.doi.org/10.1006/faat.1997.2302] [PMID: 9193927]

[38] Xiong Y, Liu Y, Cao L, *et al.* Transcriptomic Characteristics of Bronchoalveolar Lavage Fluid and Peripheral Blood Mononuclear Cells in COVID-19 Patients. Emerg Microbes Infect 2020; 9(1): 761-70.
[http://dx.doi.org/10.1080/22221751.2020.1747363]

[39] Tang X, Yin C, Zhang F, *et al.* Measurement of subgroups of peripheral blood T lymphocytes in patients with severe acute respiratory syndrome and its clinical significance. Chin Med J (Engl) 2003; 116(6): 827-30.
[PMID: 12877788]

[40] Liu X, Zhang R, He G. Hematological findings in coronavirus disease 2019: indications of progression of disease. Ann Hematol 2020; 99(7): 1421-8.
[http://dx.doi.org/10.1007/s00277-020-04103-5] [PMID: 32495027]

[41] Rajak P, Ganguly A, Sarkar S, *et al.* Immunotoxic role of organophosphates: An unseen risk escalating SARS-CoV-2 pathogenicity. Food Chem Toxicol 2021; 149: 112007.
[http://dx.doi.org/10.1016/j.fct.2021.112007] [PMID: 33493637]

[42] Zhou Y, Fu B, Zheng X, *et al.* Pathogenic T-cells and inflammatory monocytes incite inflammatory storms in severe COVID-19 patients. Natl Sci Rev 2020; 7(6): 998-1002. [http://dx.doi.org/10.1093/nsr/nwaa041] [PMID: 34676125]

[43] Blanco-Melo D, Nilsson-Payant BE, Liu WC, *et al.* Imbalanced host response to SARS-CoV-2 drives development of COVID-19. Cell 2020; 181(5): 1036-1045.e9. [http://dx.doi.org/10.1016/j.cell.2020.04.026] [PMID: 32416070]

[44] Stracke B, Rüfer C, Weibel F, *et al.* 2019; Three-Year Comparison of the Polyphenol Contents and Antioxidant Capacities in Organically and Conventionally Produced Apples (Malusdomestica Bork. Cultivar `Golden Delicious'). J Agric Food Chem 2009; 57(11): 4598-605.

[45] Zhou P, Yang XL, Wang XG, *et al.* A pneumonia outbreak associated with a new coronavirus of probable bat origin. Nature 2020; 579(7798): 270-3. [http://dx.doi.org/10.1038/s41586-020-2012-7] [PMID: 32015507]

[46] Ni L, Ye F, Cheng ML, *et al.* Detection of SARS-CoV-2-Specific Humoral and Cellular Immunity in COVID-19 Convalescent Individuals. Immunity 2020; 52(6): 971-977.e3. [http://dx.doi.org/10.1016/j.immuni.2020.04.023] [PMID: 32413330]

[47] Acharya D, Liu G, Gack MU. Dysregulation of type I interferon responses in COVID-19. Nat Rev Immunol 2020; 20(7): 397-8. [http://dx.doi.org/10.1038/s41577-020-0346-x] [PMID: 32457522]

[48] Báez-Santos YM, St John SE, Mesecar AD. The SARS-coronavirus papain-like protease: structure, function and inhibition by designed antiviral compounds. Antiviral Res 2015; 115: 21-38. [http://dx.doi.org/10.1016/j.antiviral.2014.12.015] [PMID: 25554382]

[49] Yuen CK, Lam JY, Wong WM, *et al.* SARS-CoV-2 nsp13, nsp14, nsp15 and orf6 function as potent interferon antagonists. Emerg Microbes Infect 2020; 9(1): 1418-28. [http://dx.doi.org/10.1080/22221751.2020.1780953] [PMID: 32529952]

[50] Yoshida T, Ichikawa J, Giuroiu I, *et al.* C reactive protein impairs adaptive immunity in immune cells of patients with melanoma. J Immunother Cancer 2020; 8(1): e000234. [http://dx.doi.org/10.1136/jitc-2019-000234] [PMID: 32303612]

[51] Hoffmann M, Kleine-Weber H, Schroeder S, *et al.* SARS-CoV-2 cell entry depends on ACE2 and TMPRSS2 and is blocked by a clinically proven protease inhibitor. Cell 2020; 181(2): 271-280.e8. [http://dx.doi.org/10.1016/j.cell.2020.02.052] [PMID: 32142651]

[52] Shang J, Wan Y, Luo C, *et al.* Cell entry mechanisms of SARS-CoV-2. Proc Natl Acad Sci USA 2020; 117(21): 11727-34. [http://dx.doi.org/10.1073/pnas.2003138117] [PMID: 32376634]

[53] Bajgar J. Complex view on poisoning with nerve agents and organophosphates. Acta Med (Hradec Kralove) 2005; 48(1): 3-21. [http://dx.doi.org/10.14712/18059694.2018.23] [PMID: 16080378]

[54] Namba T, Nolte CT, Jackrel J, Grob D. Poisoning due to organophosphate insecticides. Am J Med 1971; 50(4): 475-92. [http://dx.doi.org/10.1016/0002-9343(71)90337-8] [PMID: 4324629]

[55] Gagic V, Holding M, Venables WN, Hulthen AD, Schellhorn NA. Better outcomes for pest pressure, insecticide use, and yield in less intensive agricultural landscapes. Proc Natl Acad Sci USA 2021; 118(12): e2018100118. [http://dx.doi.org/10.1073/pnas.2018100118] [PMID: 33731476]

[56] Alternatives to pesticides https://www.saanich.ca/EN/main/community/natural-environment/pesticid--reduction/alternatives-to-pesticides.html

[57] Trujillo-Mayol I, Guerra-Valle M, Casas-Forero N, *et al.* Western Dietary Pattern Antioxidant Intakes and Oxidative Stress: Importance During the SARS-CoV-2/COVID-19 Pandemic. Adv Nutr 2021;

12(3): 670-81.
[http://dx.doi.org/10.1093/advances/nmaa171] [PMID: 33439972]

[58] Ahmed T, Tripathi AK, Suke SG, *et al.* Role of HSP27 and reduced glutathione in modulating malathion-induced apoptosis of human peripheral blood mononuclear cells: Ameliorating effect of N-acetylcysteine and curcumin. Toxicol In Vitro 2009; 23(7): 1319-25.
[http://dx.doi.org/10.1016/j.tiv.2009.07.016] [PMID: 19607909]

[59] Liu H, Wan Y, Wang Y, *et al.* Walnut polyphenol extract protects against fenitrothion-induced immunotoxicity in murine splenic lymphocytes. Nutrients 2018; 10(12): 1838.
[http://dx.doi.org/10.3390/nu10121838] [PMID: 30513644]

[60] Essa MM, Moghadas M, Ba-Omar T, *et al.* Protective effects of antioxidants in Huntington's disease: an extensive review. Neurotox Res 2019; 35(3): 739-74.
[http://dx.doi.org/10.1007/s12640-018-9989-9] [PMID: 30632085]

[61] Wang SY, Millner P. Effect of different cultural systems on antioxidant capacity, phenolic content, and fruit quality of strawberries (Fragaria x aranassa Duch.). J Agric Food Chem 2009; 57(20): 9651-7.
[http://dx.doi.org/10.1021/jf9020575] [PMID: 20560628]

[62] Stracke BA, Rüfer CE, Weibel FP, Bub A, Watzl B. Three-year comparison of the polyphenol contents and antioxidant capacities in organically and conventionally produced apples (Malus domestica Bork. Cultivar 'Golden Delicious'). J Agric Food Chem 2009; 57(11): 4598-605.
[http://dx.doi.org/10.1021/jf803961f] [PMID: 19388640]

CHAPTER 3

Air Quality Variation Associated with Particulate Matter in Major North Indian Cities During Diwali 2020: Susceptible Vehicle for SARS CoV-2 Transmission

Ancey Abraham[1,*] and **Insha Abbas**[2]

[1] *Department of Chemistry, Isabella Thoburn College, Lucknow-226007, India*

[2] *Department of Bioinformatics and Biotechnology, Institute of Bioinformatics and Applied Biotechnology, Bangalore-560100, India*

Abstract: Air pollution is presumed to exacerbate the COVID-19 pandemic. Previous studies have emphasized that particulate matter in the air increases the virus' infectivity and disease lethality. A study was undertaken to inspect if short-term exposure to pollutants during firecracker burning on Diwali, 2020, contributed to COVID mortality rates. Here, air quality variation was monitored concerning $PM_{2.5}$ and PM_{10} from 4th-21st November 2020 in the six most polluted cities of North India *viz.* Delhi, Lucknow, Greater Noida, Bulandshahr, Ghaziabad and Muzaffarnagar; Focussed largely on measuring pollutants' concentration pre, post and during the Diwali period, significant short-term variation in the AQI was observed during the night of Diwali which remained constant until the next day. The hazardous values recorded for AQI during the Diwali period indicated non-compliance with the ban imposed by the government on burning firecrackers in 2017. The study established a weak positive correlation between temperature and AQI, whereas a negative correlation was established between AQI and humidity. In the aftermath of the COVID-19 pandemic, short-term variations in air quality may prove to be critical.

Keywords: Air Pollution, Air Quality Variation, AQI(Air Quality Index), Correlation, COVID-19, Covid Mortality, Disease Lethality, Diwali, Exacerbate, Firecrackers, Firecracker Burning, Hazardous, Infectivity, Inspect, North India, Particulate Matter, Pollutant, Short-term Variation, Study, Virus.

INTRODUCTION

As per WHO statistics, exposure to polluted air accounts for around 4.2 million deaths every year, making it the biggest environmental health hazard. Only 1% of

* **Corresponding author Ancey Abraham:** Department of Chemistry, Isabella Thoburn College, Lucknow - 226007, India; E-mail: ancey1@gmail.com

the global population breathes air that is "good enough" in terms of quality. According to Johnson *et al.*, "Air quality is a measure of the condition of air relative to the requirements of one or more species and/or to any human need or purpose" [1]. In practice, it is estimated by the levels of major pollutants in the air *viz.* particulate matter (PM)- PM_{10}, $PM_{2.5}$, Ozone (O_3), Sulphur dioxide (SO_2), Nitrogen dioxide (NO_2), Carbon monoxide (CO), lead (Pb) and ammonia (NH_3). Air Quality Index (AQI) is a cumulative parameter for the level of these pollutants. Fig. (**1**) shows the five categories of AQI with associated health impacs. The Central Pollution Control Board (CPCB) is an organisation under the Ministry of Environment, Forest and Climate Change that routinely monitors AQI throughout India. AQI can only be calculated if sufficient data is collected; at least 6 hours of data should be available for a minimum of three pollutants. Since PM poses the most health risk, data for either PM_{10} or $PM_{2.5}$ is a mandate for this calculation. The CPCB website reports hourly AQI readings for various monitoring stations in India. The quality of air in North-Indian states has been recorded to be consistently poor, especially in the winter months. The Indian festival of Diwali falls at the onset of winter and is celebrated fervently with extravagant fireworks. The burning of firecrackers contributes to short-term spikes in AQI. Many North-Indian cities, especially in the NCR, have recorded poorly to severe AQI levels during Diwali.

AQI category	**Associated Health impact**
Good (0 to 50)	**Minimal impact**
Satisfactory (51 to 100)	**May cause minor breathing difficulties**
Moderately Polluted (101 to 200)	**May cause discomfort to people with cardiopulmonary disorders, children and the elderly**
Poor (201 to 300)	**May cause respiratory illness to people on prolonged exposure and difficulties in people with heart conditions.**
Very Poor (301 to 400)	**May cause respiratory illness to people on prolonged exposure. The effect may be more pronounced in people with lung and heart diseases.**
Severe (401 to 500)	**May cause respiratory effects even on healthy individuals and serious health impacts on people with heart/lung diseases.**

Fig. (1). Health impacts of increasing AQI values in the atmosphere.

The study of ambient air quality has become increasingly pertinent, given its implications on the COVID-19 pandemic. Numerous studies have suggested that viral transmission and COVID-19 disease progression are aided by pollutants in the air. Poor air quality not only contributes to co-morbidities in COVID-19 but also increases the risk of mortality. This chapter highlights the relationship between air pollutants and the pandemic with a special focus on particulate matter emission during the Diwali season, particulate matter *viz.* $PM_{2.5}$ and PM_{10} pose the greatest risk to health owing to their small size and deeper penetration in the lungs.

PARTICULATE MATTER: ROLE IN COVID-19

PM Exposure Increases the Risk of Developing COVID-Associated Morbidities

The pre-existence of co-morbidities significantly increases the patient's risk profile for COVID-19 infections. These include chronic cardiopulmonary disorders that are worsened by air pollution. Long-term exposure to air pollution leads to asthma, Chronic Obstructive Pulmonary Disorder (COPD), or lung fibrosis [2]. While short-term exposure may affect the respiratory system through inflammation or oxidative stress response [3]. Children are more vulnerable to these adverse effects as their lungs are still undergoing development. Their lung epithelium is also more permeable to pollutants. Poor lung development can, in turn, lead to complications in not only COVID-19 but any pulmonary disease. Overexposure to particulate matter (PM) can cause the translocation of PM into the bloodstream, where it can alter the coagulation pathway and even damage blood vessels. Reactive oxidative species (ROS) produced as a stress response have been associated with atherosclerosis, vascular dysfunction, cardiac arrhythmias and myocardial injury. The listed PM-associated comorbidities can be high-risk factors in COVID-19 patients [4].

PM can be a 'vehicle' for SARS-CoV-2 Transmission

SARS-CoV-2 is known to spread by close contact or airborne transmission. The former involves the expulsion of pathogens by infected individuals and its inhalation by the potential host. These are only effective for transmission at short distances. Another method is *via* indirect contact with infected surfaces. On the other hand, airborne transmission of the virus occurs in aerosols. Aerosol is a suspension of solid or liquid particles in the gas phase. These can be readily propagated via air currents and thus can spread infections across longer distances.

Existing research suggests that atmospheric pollutants enhance the viability of airborne pathogens [5, 6]. A study observed the spread of the avian influenza virus across long distances during storms. Correlations were drawn with the frequency of cases of measles. Another study showed similar results in context to the respiratory syncytial virus (RSV) [6]. It is hypothesized that the viral pathogens bind to particulate matter in the air, enhancing their transmissibility. Fig. (**2**) shows SARS-CoV-2 clusters deposited on $PM_{2.5}$.

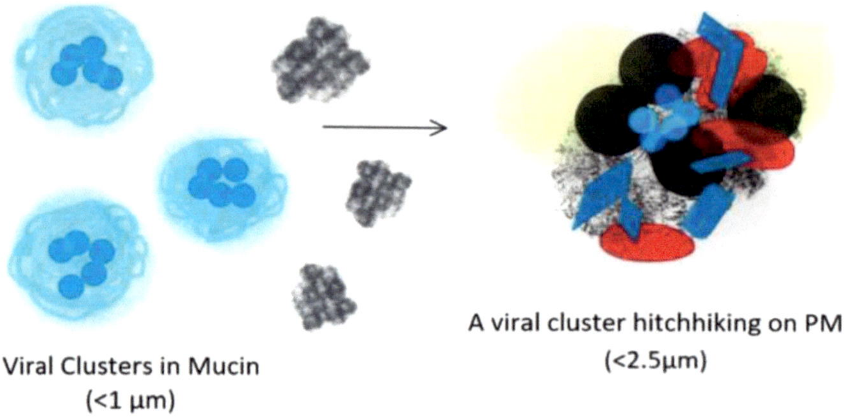

Fig. (2). Viral cluster deposition on Particulate Matter (PM).

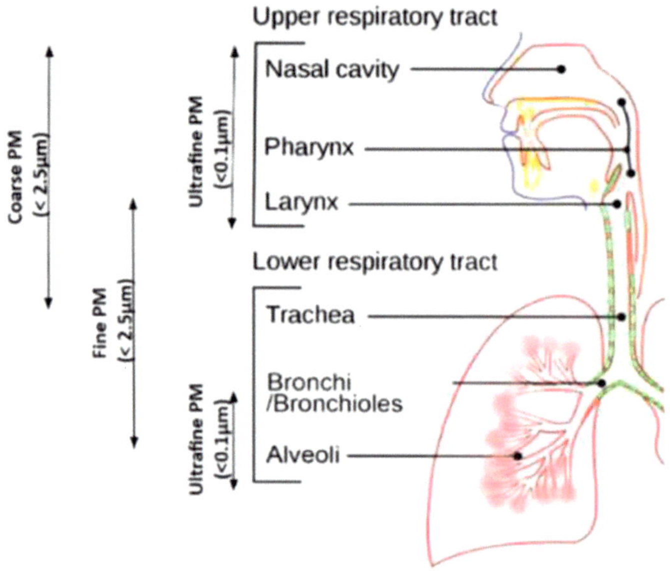

Fig. (3). Compartmental decomposition of particulate matter in the respiratory tract.

In 2020, Setti *et al.* found the first evidence of SARS-CoV-2RNA on outdoor particulate matter [7]. Findings suggest that SARS-CoV-2 can be carried from the Personal Protective Equipment (PPE) of healthcare workers by $PM_{2.5}$ in the air [8]. Another study showed that SARS-CoV-2RNA is present within particulate matter in indoor air sampling [9]. In this way, $PM_{2.5}$ poses to be another potentially infective surface. Since the size of these particles is small, they can be inhaled, and viral contact can occur directly inside the respiratory tract. Fig. (**3**) shows the compartmental deposition of PM in the respiratory tract. In addition, PM can increase viral load in individuals with less mucociliary clearance (as observed in asthma, smokers, *etc.*).

PM Increases COVID Disease Susceptibility and Severity

Angiotensin-Converting Enzyme 2 (ACE-2) is a co-receptor for the SARS-CoV-2 spike proteins. This interaction facilitates viral entry into human cells. Chronic exposure to $PM_{2.5}$ has been shown to cause overexpression of ACE-2, making the cells more vulnerable to infection [9]. Long exposures to $PM_{2.5}$ can trigger an inflammatory response. This is because ACE-2 normally has anti-inflammatory and immune functions which are blocked by the binding of the virus. A study showed that exposure to $PM_{2.5}$ induces differential expression of some genes. The viral pathogen is thought to have exploited the atmospheric environment to its advantage, as the most polluted areas are also the most populated ones. Particulate matter not only helps in rapid transmission but also aids in cell attack and entry. It weakens the immune machinery of the host and helps in disease progression. Balzo proposes this as a "synergistic co-operation" between SARS-CoV-2 and particulate matter [10].

PARTICULATE MATTER IS SUSPENDED IN THE AIR FOR LONGER IN WINTERS

The ambient air quality deteriorates during winters; the season augments the accumulation of pollutants in the atmosphere for longer. The winter season, which onsets from October and extends till February, witnesses worse air pollution due to greater suspension time of pollutants in the air, owing to the lower temperature, wind speed and high moisture content [11]. Adequate dispersion of the pollutants is hindered by these meteorological factors, resulting in frequent smog and longer retention time of pollutants at a particular place [12].

The average levels of $PM_{2.5}$ and PM_{10} are lower during the monsoon and summer seasons than during the winter [13]. The average mixing height is lower during the winter season compared to other seasons, and atmospheric dispersion is typically at a minimum, so pollutants are not as widely dispersed. Lower average mixing heights in the winter season result in less troposphere available for mixing and, as a result, higher concentrations of particulate matter. The monsoons cause a large amount of precipitation, high wind speeds, and changes in general wind direction, all of which reduce atmospheric pollution *via* associated wet deposition processes [13].

DIWALI AND THE COVID-19 PANDEMIC

There is a statistically significant increase in air pollution during Diwali [14]. The bursting of fireworks during Diwali augments the accumulation of pollutants near the surface level during winter. Hence, pollution and smog are common after Diwali, particularly in the northern part of India. The particulate matter concentration in the atmosphere that rapidly rises during the festival, results in deposition in the respiratory tract and lungs. This worsens the situation of the Covid-19 pandemic, which is primarily associated with respiratory trouble. Table **1** gives the data for COVID-19 mortality and reported cases in the city of Delhi and Lucknow. Furthermore, emissions from firecrackers during Diwali result in short-term variations in the air quality that can have long-term health effects.

The metal concentrations on the day of Diwali were found to be greater than the normal and pre-Diwali periods [15]. Both mean comparisons and correlation suggest that the burning of firecrackers on Diwali significantly contribute to air pollution with high amount of metals, especially Cu, Co, Ni, Cr and Cd, particulates (PM 2.5 and PM 10) and gaseous pollutants (SO_2 and NO_2) in the environment. The burning of firecrackers reduces the oxygen levels around since oxygen is used up in the combustion of fireworks, this could lead to the condition of asphyxiation. The metal component of firecrackers, when burnt, irritates the mucous membrane of the respiratory tract leading to excessive secretion of mucous, resulting in a cough that stays longer than usual; the cough is a reflex mechanism to expel any inhaled contaminants and to protect the respiratory tract from further damage [16].

Table 1. COVID -19 reported cases from Delhi and Lucknow.

Delhi			Lucknow		
Date	**Cases**	**Deceased**	**Date**	**Cases**	**Deceased**
04-11-2020	6842	51	04-11-2020	290	1
05-11-2020	6715	66	05-11-2020	240	11
06-11-2020	7178	64	06-11-2020	293	5
07-11-2020	6953	79	07-11-2020	241	5
08-11-2020	7745	77	08-11-2020	232	1
09-11-2020	5023	71	09-11-2020	205	2

(Table 1) cont.....

Delhi			Lucknow		
Date	**Cases**	**Deceased**	**Date**	**Cases**	**Deceased**
10-11-2020	7830	83	10-11-2020	109	4
11-11-2020	8593	85	11-11-2020	298	0
12-11-2020	7053	104	12-11-2020	315	4
13-11-2020	7802	91	13-11-2020	300	4
14-11-2020	7340	96	14-11-2020	386	2
15-11-2020	3235	95	15-11-2020	155	5
16-11-2020	3797	99	16-11-2020	247	1
17-11-2020	6396	99	17-11-2020	202	3
18-11-2020	7486	131	18-11-2020	295	6
19-11-2020	7546	98	19-11-2020	316	3
20-11-2020	6608	118	20-11-2020	400	4
21-11-2020	5879	111	21-11-2020	345	3

The Burning of Firecrackers Contributes to Air Pollution

The effect of fireworks burning during Diwali on AQI has been well established by several studies set in locations all across India [14, 15, 17]. Pratap et al., in their investigations on pollutant levels in Varanasi during Diwali, which spanned over 6 years, demonstrated that the concentrations of $PM_{2.5}$ and PM_{10} during Diwali were 5-6 times higher than the safe standard limit [14]. Similar trends have been observed in Lucknow, where the average Diwali day concentrations were up to 5 times higher than on other days [15]. Increases in trace metal concentrations in addition to PM_{10}, SO_2 and NO_2 were noted on Diwali day [15]. Another study set in Delhi found a small but significant increase in air pollution around Diwali [17].

North Indian cities are the worst-hit cities during Diwali. In 2016, the average hourly concentrations of $PM_{2.5}$ reached 910 $\mu g/m^3$, whereas the overall AQI in Delhi was observed to be severe (414) as the city was covered in toxic smog. On October 9th, 2017, the Supreme Court of India passed an order against the sale of firecrackers until the end of Diwali in Delhi and the National Capital Region (NCR). In 2018, Noida, Greater Noida and Ghaziabad were noted to have very poor AQI before Diwali, and severe AQI after the festival. Delhi in Diwali of 2019 saw concentrations up to 829.2 $\mu g/m^3$ despite the advocacy of green crackers by the Supreme Court. Consequently, bans were imposed on fireworks in Delhi, Haryana, and other states the following year. Despite this, $PM_{2.5}$ levels in Delhi and the NCR recorded a severe AQI of 469.3 $\mu g/m^3$.

The Chemistry of Fireworks

Fireworks use a specific chemical mixture that burns at the appropriate temperature, time, and with specific colours to create the brilliant patterns and forms we see. Generally, firecrackers use a substrate for burning like charcoal, manganese, *etc.*, and metal salts, such as carbonates and chlorides of lithium, barium, sodium, strontium, copper, magnesium, *etc.*, that burn with vibrant, colourful flames. Fireworks use four primary chemical elements - oxidizer, fuel, colourant and binder. Fig. (**4**) illustrates the contribution of the four main chemical elements involved in the burning of fireworks and summarizes the different colours, the metal salts produce on the burning of the firecrackers. It is these metal salts that give fireworks their different colours on burning.

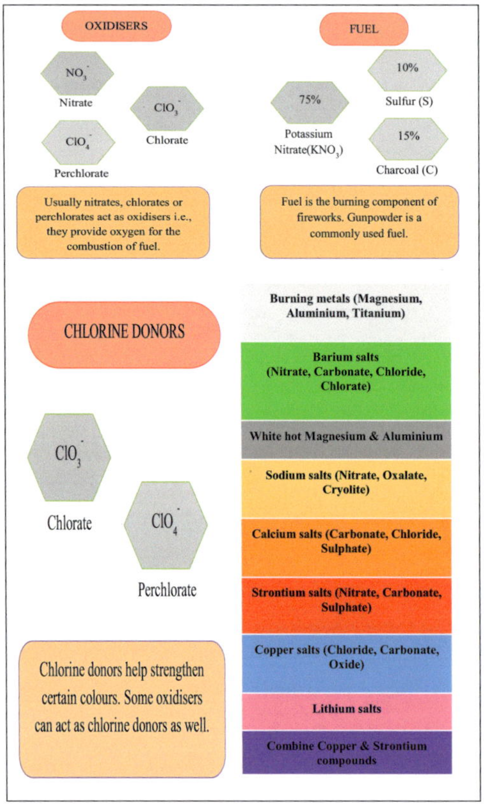

Fig. (4). The Chemistry of Fireworks [18].

Potassium perchlorate used in fireworks acts as a source of oxygen and aluminium as a source of the electron. The overall reaction is illustrated in Equation 1. Potassium perchlorate being an oxidiser aids the combustion reaction.

$$KClO_4 + Al \longrightarrow Al_2O_3 + KCl \quad \textbf{(1)}$$

Balanced form of the reaction:

$$3KClO_4 + 8Al \longrightarrow 4Al_2O_3 + 3KCl \quad \textbf{(2)}$$

The reaction in steps is as follows:

$$KClO_4 + Heat \longrightarrow KCl + O_2 \quad \textbf{(3)}$$

This reaction requires energy and hence is endergonic.

$$O_2 + Al \longrightarrow Al_2O_3 + HEAT \ \& \ LIGHT \quad \textbf{(4)}$$

This reaction releases energy as heat and light and hence is exergonic.

Fireworks emit trace gases and particles, including metals of varying sizes. Coarse particles have a mass median aerodynamic diameter (MMAD) of <10 µm, fine particles have <2.5 µm MMAD, ultrafine particles have MMAD ≤100 nm and nanoparticles have MMAD ≤50 nm. These particulates have been associated with respiratory concerns as they can travel deep into the lungs. Fig. (**5**) shows the relative size and surface area of coarse, fine and ultrafine particulate matter.

Particulate matter	**10 µm (Coarse)**	**2.5 µm (Fine)**	**0.1 µm (Ultrafine)**
Relative sizes		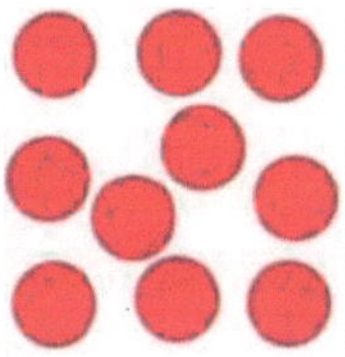	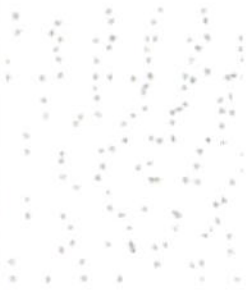
Total mass	**1**	**1**	**1**
Particle number	**1**	**64**	**10,00,000**
Total surface area per mass	**1**	**4**	**100**
Health impact	**-Filtered in proximal airway -May irritate epithelium**	**-Reaches distal airway airway -May enter the systemic circulation**	**-Adsorbs higher toxic material on the surface -May enter the systemic circulation**

Fig. (5). Relative size and surface area of coarse, fine and ultrafine particulate matter.

Firecracker Burning in a Global Context

Bursting of fireworks is a long-harboured custom, not only on the Indian festival of Diwali but in other parts of the world as well; The Chinese Lunar New Year, The Fourth of July and New Year's Day are some events that are celebrated with fireworks every year. Extensive firecracker burning has serious environmental concerns and associated health hazards. Last year, Beijing and North China were blanketed in heavy smog for 3 consecutive days following the celebrations [19]. Los Angeles County air pollution levels, soared up to 10 times higher than average on July 4, 2020 [20]. Burns, injuries, and fires in buildings or forests are common occurrences during these festivities.

IMPACT ON AIR QUALITY VARIATION AND HEALTH DURING DIWALI 2020: A CASE STUDY

Material and Methods

A study was conducted to assess the impact of firecracker burning during the Diwali festival on air pollution in the six most polluted cities of North India. These six cities were categorized as "very poor" in terms of AQI at the onset of the winter season in 2020 by the Central Pollution Control Board [12]. The main aim of the study was to monitor air quality variation because of firecracker burning and the impact of meteorological factors like temperature, humidity and wind speed on the AQI, and if daily variation in the AQI had any relation with the COVID-19 cases reported in these particular cities during the study period.

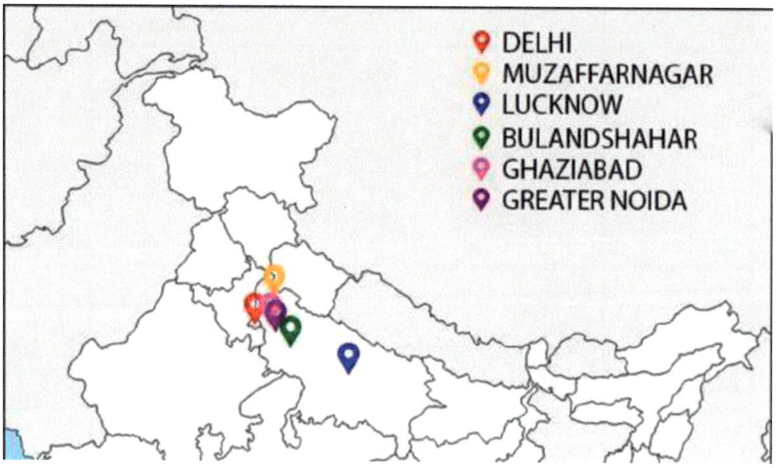

Fig. (6). Northern region of India with the six selected cities.

For the assessment, the variation in AQI was recorded for $PM_{2.5}$ and PM_{10} from 4th - 21st November 2020 in intervals of 3 hours, *i.e.*, at 8 a.m., 11 a.m., 2 p.m., 5 p.m., 10 p.m., and 12 a.m. Since the present study was focused on measuring pollutants' concentration pre, post and during Diwali to assess short-term variation and its health impacts, hourly variations in the AQI, *i.e.*, from 6 a.m. to 12 a.m., were recorded from 12th-16th November 2020. The data was recorded from www.aqicn.org and the AQI values were converted into concentration to determine the average concentration of the pollutants using an online calculator at www.airnow.gov. The COVID-19 cases reported during the study period were also taken into account. Fig. (**6**) shows the northern part of India with the six selected cities.

Results and Discussion

A record of the average concentration of $PM_{2.5}$ and PM_{10} from 10th November 2020 - 17th November 2020 during the study period (4th - 21st Nov, 2020) is accounted for in Table **2** and represented in (Fig. **7**). The AQI values were converted using an online AQI to concentration converter. AQI values greater than 500 could not be converted and hence were not taken into consideration during analysis. Delhi, Lucknow and Bulandshahr recorded their highest PM 2.5 concentrations (µg/m^3) on the day of Diwali, *i.e.*, 14th November 2020 as 412, 337 and 520, respectively, whereas Ghaziabad (482), Greater Noida (456) and Muzaffarnagar (292) recorded their highest during the pre-Diwali period. The highest PM 10 concentrations(µg/m^3) recorded for Delhi, Lucknow, Bulandshahr, Ghaziabad, Greater Noida and Muzaffarnagar, were 565, 572, 548, 532, 586 and 587, respectively, all in the pre- Diwali period. The lowest concentrations were recorded between 16th-17th November when North India received heavy rainfall between 3.1-4.4 mm, which could be responsible for the wash-out effect [12].

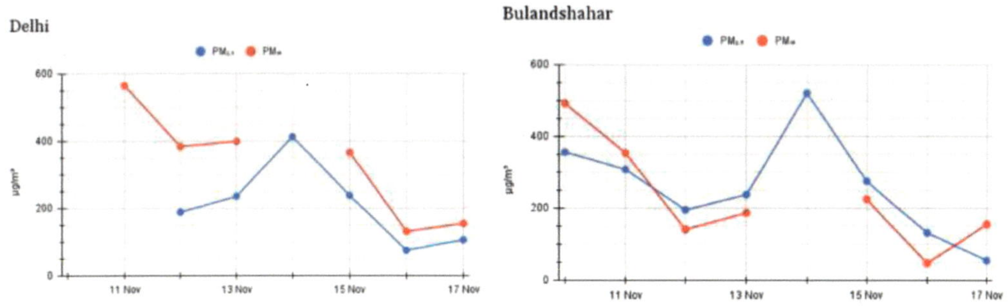

(Fig. 7) contd.....

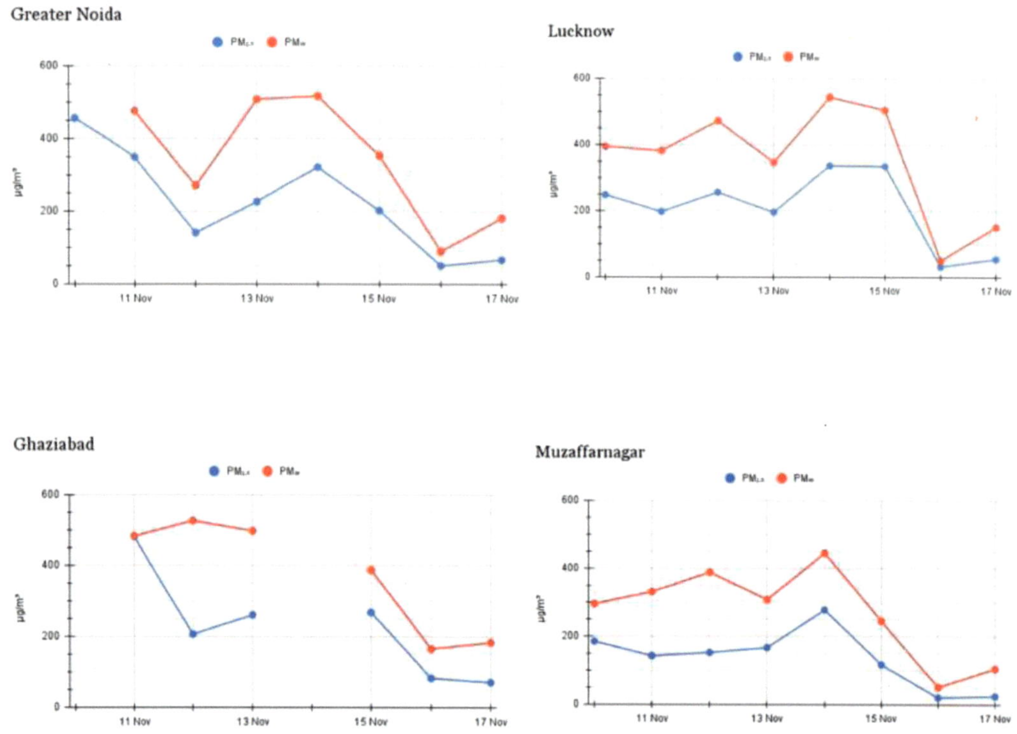

Fig. (7). Average Concentration of $PM_{2.5}$ and PM_{10} during Diwali, 2020.

Table 2. Average Concentration of $PM_{2.5}$ and PM_{10} in the six cities from 10th-17th November 2020.

	DELHI		LUCKNOW		BULANDSHAHAR	
Date	**$PM_{2.5}$ (µg/m³)**	**PM_{10} (µg/m³)**	**$PM_{2.5}$ (µg/m³)**	**PM_{10} (µg/m³)**	**$PM_{2.5}$ (µg/m³)**	**PM_{10} (µg/m³)**
10/11/20	NA	NA	248	394	356.5	492
11/11/20	NA	565	198	382	308	354
12/11/20	187.8	384	256	472	195.14	140.7
13/11/20	235.2	399	196	347	237.32	186.8
14/11/20	412.5	NA	337	543	520	NA
15/11/20	237.2	366	335	504	275	225.1
16/11/20	74.8	131	32	50	131.38	47.6
17/11/20	105.8	154	55	151	55	155

(Table 2) cont.....

	GHAZIABAD		GREATER NOIDA		MUZAFFARNAGAR	
Date	**PM $_{2.5}$ (µg/m^3)**	**PM $_{10}$ (µg/m^3)**	**PM $_{2.5}$ (µg/m^3)**	**PM $_{10}$ (µg/m^3)**	**PM $_{2.5}$ (µg/m^3)**	**PM $_{10}$ (µg/m^3)**
10/11/20	NA	NA	456.4	NA	184.8	295
11/11/20	482.2	482	349.3	476	142.6	331
12/11/20	206	526	140.7	271	152.5	389
13/11/20	260.5	497	226.1	508	166.6	308
14/11/20	NA	NA	322.1	517	277.7	445
15/11/20	267.6	387	201.9	354	117.4	245
16/11/20	82.6	165	50.5	90	20.6	51
17/11/20	70.9	183	67.1	181	24.4	105

Short-Term Exposure

Ravindra *et al.* (2003) reported that the burning of firecrackers during Diwali leads to a short-term variation in the air quality with a 2-3 times increased concentration of PM_{10}. Short-term exposure can have long-term effects and has also been associated with adverse health effects and mortality rates. Due to the fireworks, around 30-40% increase in the cases of wheezing, respiratory infections, and exacerbation of bronchial asthma has been reported during Diwali [21]. Hospitalization due to respiratory problems post-Diwali has been reported to be more than pre-Diwali in both rural and urban areas [22]. Table **3** summarizes the short-term effects of $PM_{2.5}$ and $PM_{10,}$ along with their threshold limits.

Table 3. 24-hour threshold limits of $PM_{2.5}$ and PM_{10} and their short-term effects.

Pollutant	**WHO Limit (µg/m^3)**	**Short Term Effect**
$PM_{2.5}$	25	Lung irritation, coughing, sneezing, runny nose and shortness of breath
PM_{10}	50	Cardiac and respiratory-related hospitalizations

It has been observed that an elevation in the concentration of pollutants leads to an inflammatory response, including alveolar cytokine release, which is responsible for bronchospasm and impaired pulmonary infection [22]. Short-term exposure to elevated concentrations of trace elements from fireworks can cause neurological and haematological effects on the exposed population [23].

The observed AQI values were quite poor throughout the day of Diwali and were mostly in the 'hazardous category', with AQI deteriorating after 6 p.m. Table **4** accounts for the hourly variations in AQI for $PM_{2.5}$ and PM_{10} for the six cities recorded from 6 a.m. to 12 a.m. in the night on the day of Diwali. The maximum

AQI values reported for the cities of Delhi, Lucknow, Bulandshahr, Ghaziabad, Greater Noida and Muzaffarnagar for $PM_{2.5}$ were 530, 690, 999, 706, 520, 824, respectively and for PM_{10} were 854, 999, 999, 999, 618, 999 respectively. All six cities were observed to have constant AQI after 9 p.m. and reached the highest around midnight and remained so till the next morning. Fig. (**8**) represents the hourly variation in AQI in the six cities as recorded on the day of Diwali for $PM_{2.5.}$

Table 4. Hourly variations in AQI for $PM_{2.5}$ and PM_{10} for the six cities recorded from 6 a.m. to 12 a.m. in the night on the day of Diwali.

DELHI			LUCKNOW (LALBAGH)		GHAZIABAD	
TIME	$PM_{2.5}$	PM_{10}	$PM_{2.5}$	PM_{10}	$PM_{2.5}$	PM_{10}
6:00 a.m.	434	372	188	117	502	530
7:00 a.m.	434	372	191	130	502	550
8:00 a.m.	496	469	195	134	539	662
9:00 a.m.	492	495	195	139	539	662
10:00 a.m.	492	495	217	157	513	684
11:00 a.m.	535	646	202	145	513	684
12:00 a.m.	514	593	191	143	534	732
1:00 a.m.	464	531	184	129	534	732
2:00 a.m.	464	531	175	138	534	732
3:00 a.m.	340	296	175	138	534	732
4:00 a.m.	217	139	171	108	267	209
5:00 a.m.	223	138	187	114	302	338
6:00 a.m.	244	168	206	135	428	654
7:00 a.m.	307	225	223	151	500	841
8:00 a.m.	442	537	317	422	500	841
9:00 a.m.	530	697	379	454	544	765
10:00 a.m.	530	824	490	764	706	970
11:00 a.m.	530	824	690	999	706	999
12:00 a.m.	530	854	731	999	706	999
BULANDSHAHAR			MUZAFFARNAGAR		GREATER NOIDA	
TIME	$PM_{2.5}$	PM_{10}	$PM_{2.5}$	PM_{10}	$PM_{2.5}$	PM_{10}
6:00 a.m.	432	403	317	177	402	357
7:00 a.m.	427	402	317	178	430	451
8:00 a.m.	418	394	317	181	460	506
9:00 a.m.	430	432	317	218	462	552

(Table 4) cont.....

10:00 a.m.	516	585	317	273	420	490
11:00 a.m.	395	387	276	192	417	461
12:00 a.m.	377	392	263	178	406	448
1:00 a.m.	329	266	206	121	315	293
2:00 a.m.	310	230	163	81	258	180
3:00 a.m.	213	156	163	74	213	152
4:00 a.m.	248	178	154	64	195	138
5:00 a.m.	273	354	176	120	218	237
6:00 a.m.	317	417	188	153	246	499
7:00 a.m.	541	973	221	200	323	456
8:00 a.m.	775	999	298	470	412	472
9:00 a.m.	999	999	376	563	414	471
10:00 a.m.	999	999	744	999	456	493
11:00 a.m.	999	999	824	999	493	578
12:00 a.m.	829	975	650	999	520	618

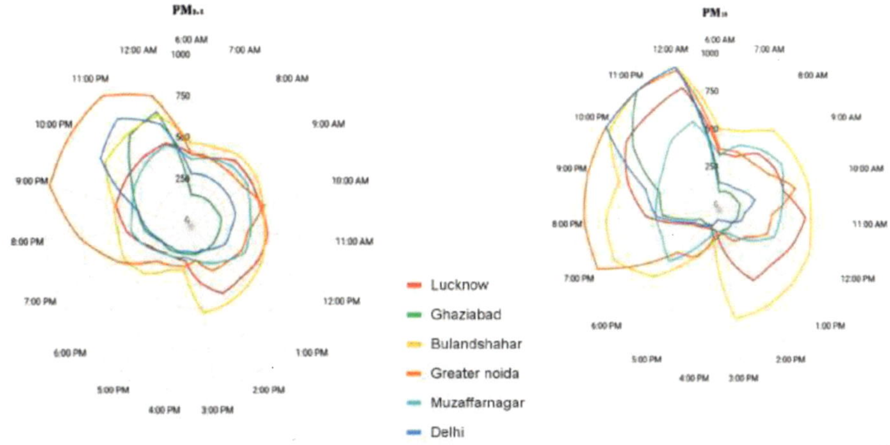

Fig. (8). Hourly variation in AQI for $PM_{2.5}$ and PM_{10}.

Meteorological Parameters and their Effect on AQI

The fate of the air pollutants is influenced by the air movements, *i.e.*, when the air is still, proper diffusion of the pollutants does not occur, and their concentration builds up. On the other hand, due to strong and turbulent winds, quick dispersion of pollutants takes place, resulting in lower concentrations. Hence, meteorological parameters such as temperature, wind speed and relative humidity play a vital role in the dispersion of pollutants.

To study the correlation between AQI and meteorological parameters, average temperature, humidity and wind speed were recorded for the six selected cities during the study period. Table **5** gives the data for the meteorological parameters and (Figs. **9** and **10**) represent the correlation between Temperature and Relative humidity with AQI, respectively.

Table 5. Meteorological data for the 6 selected cities.

City	Average Temperature (°C)	Average Humidity	Average Wind Speed (Km/h)
Lucknow	21.96±1.48	57.30±12.88	2.47±2.25
Muzaffarnagar	30.65±1.22	48.50±11.25	1.38±1.02
Greater Noida	32.96±0.46	46.51±12.36	2.13±0.73
Bulandshahar	32.45±0.65	46.75±6.23	2.50±1.58
Ghaziabad	29.01±0.43	63.71	4.51±1.83
New Delhi	19.16±2.91	66.51±0.35	0.97±1.26

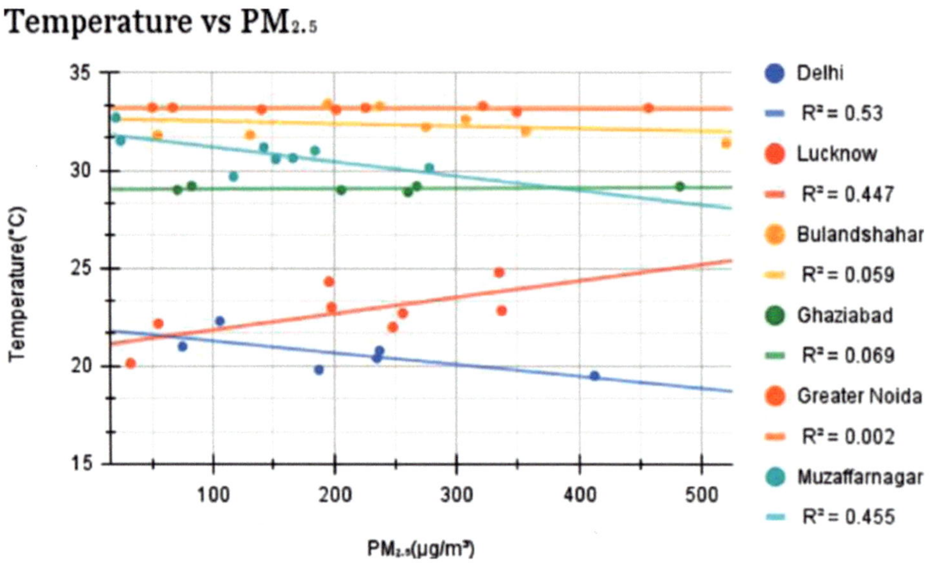

Fig. (9). Correlation between Temperature and AQI for $PM_{2.5}$.

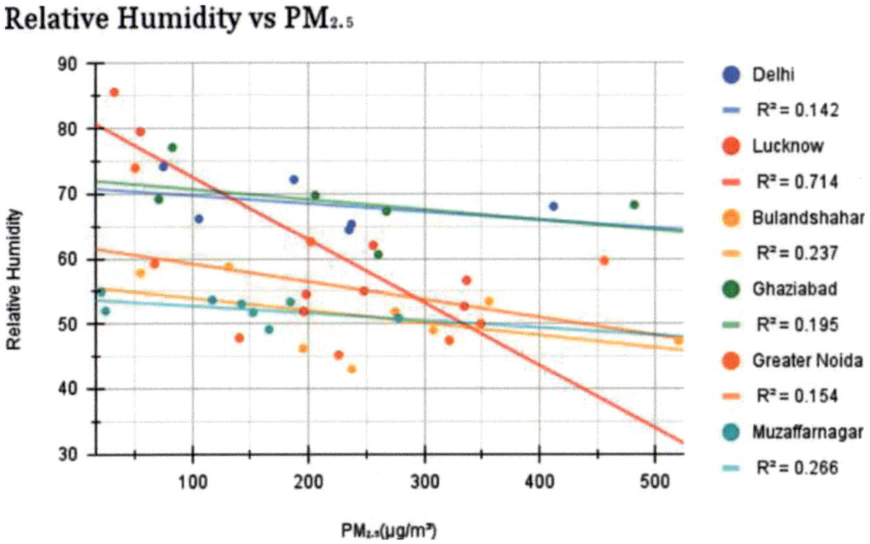

Fig. (10). Correlation between Relative humidity and AQI for $PM_{2.5}$.

A weak positive correlation was observed between temperature and $PM_{2.5,}$ whereas a negative correlation was observed for humidity. The negative correlation for humidity could be due to the increase in the rate of absorption of particulate matter with the increase in humidity. The adsorption of SARS-CoV-2 on the particulate matter can result in long-range transportation, ultimately leading to higher transmission probability. A study conducted in the United States linked $PM_{2.5}$ levels to mortality rates, concluding that countries with high annual particulate contamination, such as India, are more vulnerable [12]. Also, according to a study in Italy, the virus became more lethal in high-pollution areas such as Lombardy and Emilia Romagna, making it an important co-factor [12].

RESPIRATORY HEALTH AROUND THE GLOBE

More than 10% of all disability-adjusted life-years (DALYs), a statistic that reflects the amount of active and productive life lost owing to an illness, are attributable to respiratory disorders. According to WHO estimates [24], 65 million people worldwide suffer from moderate to severe chronic obstructive pulmonary disease (COPD), with around 3 million dying each year, making it the third greatest cause of mortality. Asthma affects around 334 million people worldwide, and it is the most prevalent chronic illness in childhood, impacting 14% of children. In 2020, 1.5 million individuals will have perished from tuberculosis. TB is the world's 13th biggest cause of mortality and the second leading infectious killer after COVID-19. COPD is third, lower respiratory tract infection is fourth, tracheal, bronchial, and lung cancer is sixth, tuberculosis is twelfth, and asthma is twenty-eighth among the top 30 causes of mortality. According to a study [25], in 2016, India accounted for 32.0 percent of all worldwide DALYs attributable to chronic respiratory illnesses. COPD and asthma accounted for 75.6 percent and 20.0 percent of the chronic respiratory illness DALYs, respectively. From 1990 to 2016, the number of cases of COPD in India increased from 3.3 percent to 4.2 percent. Tobacco use was responsible for 25.4 percent of DALYs, occupational hazards for 16.5 percent, and air pollution was the leading cause with 53.7 percent.

CONCLUSION

As depicted by the average particulate matter concentration and hourly variation data, the fireworks were found to be responsible for elevated concentrations during the Diwali period. In a time when respiratory trouble is at its peak and causing a threat to human lives due to the Covid-19 pandemic, it is only prudent to discourage the burning of firecrackers. Despite the ban imposed on the burning of firecrackers, hazardous AQI values were recorded from Delhi, Lucknow, Ghaziabad, Bulandshahr, Muzaffarnagar and Greater Noida, the six cities selected for the study. Those with underlying chronic lung and cardiovascular diseases are more prone to infection during Diwali, hence, exposure to massive bursts of short-term variation in the air quality can also lead to significant short-term and long-term health effects. The present study did not suggest any positive correlation between the Covid-19 related cases and the deterioration of the AQI in short-term exposure. However, long-term exposure to air pollution along with Covid-19 infection can have chronic health effects

CONSENT FOR PUBLICATION

Not applicable.

CONFLICT OF INTEREST

The authors declare no conflict of interest, financial or otherwise.

ACKNOWLEDGEMENTS

The authors extend the acknowledgements to Dr. (Mrs.) V. Prakash, The Principal, Isabella Thoburn College, Lucknow, for their support.

REFERENCES

[1] Johnson DL, Ambrose SH, Bassett TJ, *et al.* Meanings of Environmental Terms. J Environ Qual 1997; 26(3): 581-9. [http://dx.doi.org/10.2134/jeq1997.00472425002600030002x]

[2] Bourdrel T, Maesano I, Allahmad B, Maesno C N, Bind M. The impact of outdoor air pollution on

COVID-19: a review of evidence from in vitro, animal, and human studies Eur Respir review 2021; 30: 0242-2020.

[3] Chen Z, Huang BZ, Sidell MA, *et al.* Near-roadway air pollution associated with COVID-19 severity and mortality – Multiethnic cohort study in Southern California. Environ Int 2021; 157106862. [http://dx.doi.org/10.1016/j.envint.2021.106862] [PMID: 34507232]

[4] Du Y, Xu X, Chu M. et al. Air particulate matter and cardiovascular disease: the epidemiological, biomedical and clinical evidence. J Thorac Dis 2016; 8(1): 8-19.

[5] Noda J, Tomizawa S, Takahashi K, Morimoto K, Mitarai S. Air pollution and airborne infection with mycobacterial bioaerosols: a potential attribution of soot. Int J Environ Sci Technol 2021; 1-10. [PMID: 33643419]

[6] Comunian S, Dongo D, Milani C, Palestini P. Air Pollution and COVID-19: The Role of Particulate Matter in the Spread and Increase of COVID-19's Morbidity and Mortality. Int J Environ Res Public Health 2020; 17(12): 4487. [http://dx.doi.org/10.3390/ijerph17124487] [PMID: 32580440]

[7] Setti L, Passarini F, De Gennaro G, *et al.* SARS-Cov-2RNA found on particulate matter of Bergamo in Northern Italy: First evidence. Environ Res 2020; 188: 109754. [http://dx.doi.org/10.1016/j.envres.2020.109754] [PMID: 32526492]

[8] Ong SWX, Tan YK, Chia PY, *et al.* Air, surface environmental, and personal protective equipment contamination by severe acute respiratory syndrome coronavirus 2 (SARS-CoV-2) from a symptomatic patient. JAMA 2020; 323(16): 1610-2. [http://dx.doi.org/10.1001/jama.2020.3227] [PMID: 32129805]

[9] Frontera A, Cianfanelli L, Vlachos K, Landoni G, Cremona G. Severe air pollution links to higher mortality in COVID-19 patients: The "double-hit" hypothesis. J Infect 2020; 81(2): 255-9. [http://dx.doi.org/10.1016/j.jinf.2020.05.031] [PMID: 32447007]

[10] Balzo G. Energy Landscape Theory of SARS-CoV-2 Complexes with Particulate Matter. SSRN 2020. [http://dx.doi.org/10.2139/ssrn.3609572]

[11] Lawrence A, Fatima N. Impact of firecrackers on indoor air in Diwali festival in Lucknow city- The second largest city of North India. Indian J Environ Protect 2014; 34(8).

[12] Lawrence AJ, Abraham A, Ali F, *et al.* Air Quality in Six Northern Indian Cities During Diwali 2020: The Real Tragedy in Disguise. Asian J Chem 2021; 33(4): 909-18. [http://dx.doi.org/10.14233/ajchem.2021.23102]

[13] Pandey P, Khan AH, Verma AK, *et al.* Seasonal trends of PM2.5 and PM10 in ambient air and their correlation in ambient air of Lucknow city, India. Bull Environ Contam Toxicol 2012; 88(2): 265-70. [http://dx.doi.org/10.1007/s00128-011-0466-x] [PMID: 22105933]

[14] Pratap V, Saha U, Kumar A, Singh AK. Analysis of air pollution in the atmosphere due to firecrackers in the Diwali period over an urban Indian region. Adv Space Res 2021; 68(8): 3327-41. [http://dx.doi.org/10.1016/j.asr.2021.06.031]

[15] Barman SC, Singh R, Negi MPS, Bhargava SK. Ambient air quality of Lucknow City (India) during use of fireworks on Diwali Festival. Environ Monit Assess 2008; 137(1-3): 495-504. [http://dx.doi.org/10.1007/s10661-007-9784-1] [PMID: 17562206]

[16] Keerthana P, Sundar N, Ananda Kumar S. Fireworks in times of COVID-19: A Predictable disaster. International Journal of Advanced Research in Science. Int J Adv Res Sci 2020; 9(1): 89-91.

[17] Ghei D, Sane R. Estimates of air pollution in Delhi from the burning of firecrackers during the festival of Diwali. PLoS One 2018; 13(8): e0200371. [http://dx.doi.org/10.1371/journal.pone.0200371] [PMID: 30102708]

[18] Limaye S, Shah R, Ujagare D, Madas S, Salvi S, Salvi S. Personal exposures to particulate matter <2.5 μm in mass median aerodynamic diameter ($PM_{2.5}$) pollution during the burning of six most commonly

used firecrackers in India. Lung India 2019; 36(4): 324-9.
[http://dx.doi.org/10.4103/lungindia.lungindia_440_18] [PMID: 31290418]

[19] Weather.com [homepage on the Internet]. Air Pollution Remains High in Beijing Post Chinese New Year; 2021 [posted on 15th February, 2021.] Available from: https://weather.com/en-IN/india/pollution/news/2021-02-15-air-pollution-remains-high-in-beijing-post-chinese-new-year

[20] [homepage on the Internet].The hidden toll of July Fourth fireworks; 2021 [posted on 2nd July 2021] Available from: https://www.nationalgeographic.com/environment/article/the-hidden-toll-of--uly-fourth-fireworksnationalgeographic.com

[21] Chatterjee A, Sarkar C, Adak A, Mukherjee U, Ghosh SK, Raha S. Ambient Air Quality during Diwali Festival over Kolkata - A Mega-City in India. Aerosol Air Qual Res 2013; 13(3): 1133-44.
[http://dx.doi.org/10.4209/aaqr.2012.03.0062]

[22] Pope CA III, Dockery DW. Health effects of fine particulate air pollution: lines that connect. J Air Waste Manag Assoc 2006; 56(6): 709-42.
[http://dx.doi.org/10.1080/10473289.2006.10464485] [PMID: 16805397]

[23] Ghio AJ, Kim C, Devlin RB. Concentrated ambient air particles induce mild pulmonary inflammation in healthy human volunteers. Am J Respir Crit Care Med 2000; 162(3): 981-8.
[http://dx.doi.org/10.1164/ajrccm.162.3.9911115] [PMID: 10988117]

[24] Forum of International Respiratory Societies, Sheffield, European Respiratory Society. The Global Impact of Respiratory Disease – Second Edition 2017; 7-8.

[25] Salvi S, Kumar GA, Dhaliwal RS, *et al.* The burden of chronic respiratory diseases and their heterogeneity across the states of India: the Global Burden of Disease Study 1990–2016. Lancet Glob Health 2018; 6(12): e1363-74.
[http://dx.doi.org/10.1016/S2214-109X(18)30409-1] [PMID: 30219316]

CHAPTER 4

COVID-19 and Moderating Effects of Government Stimulus

Mehul Raithatha[1,*] and **Robinson Reyes-Peña**[2]

[1] *Finance and Accounting Area, Indian Institute of Management, Indore, India*

[2] *Department of Finance, College of Business Administration, Florida International University, Miami, FL, USA*

Abstract: In this paper, we study the impact of the COVID-19 pandemic on the economic conditions and the stock markets of countries across the world. We find that an increase in contagion and death rate due to the pandemic inversely affects both the country's GDP and its stock markets. Next, we study the impact of government stimulus on the economic conditions and the stock markets of each of the countries in our sample. We find that the government stimulus moderates the effect of COVID-19 on the real condition of economies as we find that GDP is not affected by COVID-1--related death in the post-stimulus period. The stimulus alleviates the negative impact of pandemic concerns on the stock markets, where the increase in contagion and death rate due to COVID-19 positively correlates with the performance of stock markets in the post-stimulus period.

Keywords: COVID-19, Government Stimulus, Pandemic, Post-stimulus, Stock Market Performance.

INTRODUCTION

COVID-19 pandemic started spreading worldwide early in the year 2020, and countries faced the dilemma of closing day-to-day activities to minimize social interactions to contain the contagion and death rate and suffer economic suicide or continuing social activities to protect their economies. The increased death rates due to COVID-19 consequently imposed social distancing measures in most of the countries in order to control the spread and death due to COVID-19. In this paper, we study the impact of pandemic contagion and death rates on the real economic conditions of countries and their stock markets. We find that increase in contagion and death rate due to the pandemic inversely affects both, the stock markets as well as the country's GDP.

* **Corresponding author Mehul Raithatha**: Finance and Accounting Area, Indian Institute of Management, Indore, India; E-mail: mehulr@iimidr.ac.in

Alfred J. Lawrence & Tahmeena Khan (Eds.)

To alleviate the economic fallouts, countries across the world enacted laws providing a significant amount of money in their economies. We study the impact of government stimulus on the economic conditions and the stock markets of each of the countries in our sample. We find that stimulus alleviates the pandemic concerns for the stock markets, where an increase in contagion and death rate due to COVID-19 has a positive correlation with the performance of stock markets in the post-stimulus period. The government stimulus moderates the effect of COVID-19 on real economic conditions as well. We find no relationship between the GDP and the increase in contagion and death rate in the post-stimulus period.

The literature on the effect of COVID-19 on global economies is in a developmental stage where several researchers have shown a negative effect of COVID-19 spread on the global economies and their stock markets. A study [1] conducted in the early days of the pandemic from January 22 to April 17, 2020, found that an increase in COVID-19 cases and deaths has a negative effect on stock prices across the world. They find that the stock market reaction is more severe for the increase in the number of cases than the number of deaths. Another study by the same author [2] finds that government social distancing measures in response to COVID-19 have a direct negative effect on stock markets across the world due to their adverse effect on economic activities. Erdem (2020) [3] found that COVID-19 has a significantly negative effect on stock markets across the world, but the adverse effect on stock markets are less severe in freer countries. Zhang *et al.* (2020) [4] analyze country-specific risk and systematic risks of the global financial markets in response to COVID-19 and discuss the potential consequences of governmental response to mitigate COVID-19 spread. They find a negative effect of COVID-19 spread on global stock markets. Haroon *et al.* (2020) [5] find an increase in stock market volatility due to the COVID-19-related news. Mazur *et al.* (2020) [6] investigated the performance of the US stock market during March 2020 and found that negative response is severe in petroleum, real estate, entertainment and hospitality sectors, whereas food, healthcare and technology stocks show positive returns in the COVID-19 crisis. Goodell (2020) [7] provides an agenda for future research related to COVID-19 and finance. Our paper investigates two of the six research areas suggested by Goodell (2020) [7]. He points out the need for research to explore the economic impact of the pandemic and to study the impact of pandemics on financial markets.

In this paper, we contribute to the literature by formally testing the impact of government stimulus on the real economic conditions and the stock market performance of countries across the world. Using the stock market index and GDP data for a sample of 18 countries, we confirm an inverse relation between COVID-19 cases and death rates on the stock markets across the world. Our choice of countries depends on the availability of index-related data on yahoo finance. Our empirical analysis shows that the negative effect of COVID-19 cases and deaths on the GDP and stock markets is alleviated by the government stimulus.

DATA AND METHODOLOGY

We use Yahoo finance for daily stock market index data which is available for 18 countries (see Appendix 1). When multiple index data is available for a particular country, we choose only one major stock index from the sample country. We use the data of daily COVID-19 confirmed cases and deaths for each country from the John Hopkins University, Coronavirus Resource Centre website. The GDP data is from the OECD website. Our sample period is from January 23 to August 18, 2020, which allows us to adequately cover the period from the start of COVID-19 in each sample country to the post-stimulus period. To capture the effects of culture, we use Hofstede's (2001) [8] six dimensions [https://geerthofstede.com/research-and-vsm/dimension-data-matrix/] and to capture the role of institutions, we use the latest scores from the International Country Risk Guide (ICRG)[https://www.prsgroup.com/explore-our-products/international-country-risk-guide/]. For economic activity measurement, we collect quarterly GDP data for the first and second quarters of 2020. We have 34 observations for the first and second quarters for GDP analysis. To study the impact of COVID-19 on GDP, we use the following model.

$$GDP\_Change_{c,q} = \propto_c + \beta_1\, COVID19_{c,q} + \beta_c\, Country_{FE} + \varepsilon_{c,t} \quad (1)$$

Where c and q subscripts represent the country and quarter, respectively. α_c is the constant term, and $E_{c,g}$ is the error term. $COVID19_{c,q}$ represents $COVID19\_Cases_q$ *per million* and $COVID19\_Death_t$ per million in separate models. To test the moderating effect of fiscal stimulus, we use the following model.

$$GDP\_Change_{c,q} = \propto_c + \beta_1\, COVID19_{q,t} + \beta_2 Fiscal\ Stimulus\ Dummy_c + \beta_3 COVID-19_{q,t} * Fiscal\ Stimulus\ Dummy_c + \beta_c\, Country_{FE} + + \varepsilon_{c,t} \quad (2)$$

Where *Financial Stimulus Dummy* takes a value of one for the post-stimulus period (quarter 2 of 2020) for each of the countries in our sample and zero (quarter 1 of 2020) otherwise. The interaction term captures the effect of COVID-19 on GDP in the post-stimulus period.

To study the impact of the pandemic on the stock market performance, we use daily data on the stock market index and COVID-19 infections. We generate the following variables on a daily basis (where *t* subscript represents day).

$$Index\_Return_t = (Index\_Value_t - Index\_Value_{t-1})/Index\_Value_{t-1}$$

$$COVID19\_Death\_rate_t = (deaths\ per\ million_t - deaths\ per\ million_{t-1})/deaths\ per\ million_{t-1}$$

$$COVID19\_infection\_rate_t = (cases\ per\ million_t - cases\ per\ million_{t-1})/cases\ per\ million_{t-1}$$

Using the index return and the COVID-19 infection rate and death rate, we run the following regression equation to test our third hypothesis.

$$Index_{Return\,c,t} = \propto_c + \beta_1\ COVID19_{c,t} + \beta_c\ Country_{FE} + \varepsilon_{c,t} \quad (3)$$

Where c and t subscripts represent country and day respectively. α_c is the constant term and $\varepsilon_{c,t}$ is the error term. $COVID19_{c,t}$ represents $COVID19\_infection\_rate_t$ and $COVID19\_death\_rate_t$ in separate models. To test the moderating effect of fiscal stimulus, we use the following model.

$$Index\_Return_{c,t} = \propto_c + \beta_1\ COVID19_{c,t} + \beta_2 Fiscal\ Stimulus\ Dummy_c + \beta_3 COVID19_{c,t} * Fiscal\ Stimulus\ Dummy_c + \beta_c\ Country_{FE} + \varepsilon_{c,t} \quad (4)$$

Where *Financial Stimulus Dummy* takes a value of one for the post-stimulus period for each of the countries in our sample and zeroes otherwise. The interaction term captures the effect of COVID-19 on the stock market returns in the post-stimulus period.

RESULTS

Impact of COVID on Real Economy: Moderating Effect of Fiscal Stimulus

In Table **1,** we provide the descriptive statistics for the change in GDP of the countries in our sample and the COVID-19 cases and deaths per million in these countries. We find an average decrease of 5.1% in GDP per quarter, an average of 1266 cases per million, and an average of 108 deaths per million per quarter. This table reports the summary statistics of variables used in our GDP analysis.

Table 1. Descriptive statistics for GDP analysis (N=34).

Variable	Mean	Std. Dev.	Minimum	Maximum
Change in GDP	-5.10	5.97	-20.37	11.50
Death per million	107.60	199.96	0.00	831.00
Cases per million	1265.83	1998.18	0.91	7826.38

In (Fig. **1a),** we plot the scatter graph and trendline for the change in GDP and the death per million, and in (Fig. **1d)** we provide a similar plot for the change in GDP and the number of cases per million. The negative slope of the trendline indicates a decrease in GDP for the increase in COVID-19 cases and deaths. In (Figs. **1b and 1c),** we separately plot the graph in (Fig. **1a**) for deaths related to COVID-19 in Quarter 1 and for Quarter 2, respectively. Similarly, in (Figs. **1e** and **1f**), we plot separate graphs for quarter 1 and quarter 2 for the number of COVID-19 cases. We notice a steeper slope in the second quarter, indicating a more severe effect of COVID-19 cases and deaths on GDP in the second quarter of 2020.

In (Figs. **2a and 2b**), we plot the marginal effects of COVID-19 cases and deaths on GDP in quarters 1 and quarter 2. The marginal effect for the number of deaths reduces in the post-stimulus period, and the marginal effects stay the same in quarter2 for the number of cases indicating the moderating effect of stimulus in containing the impact of COVID-19 on the GDP of countries in our sample.

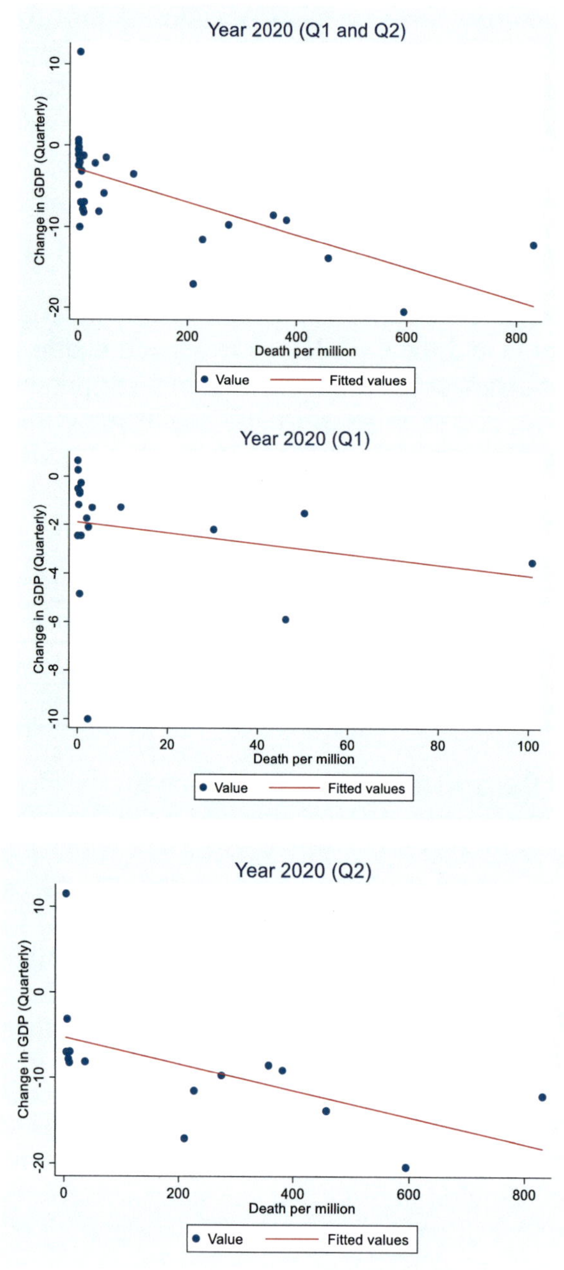
Year 2020 (Q1 and Q2)
Change in GDP (Quarterly)
Death per million
Value
Fitted values
Year 2020 (Q1)
Change in GDP (Quarterly)
Death per million
Value
Fitted values
Year 2020 (Q2)
Change in GDP (Quarterly)
Death per million
Value
Fitted values

(Fig. 1) contd.....

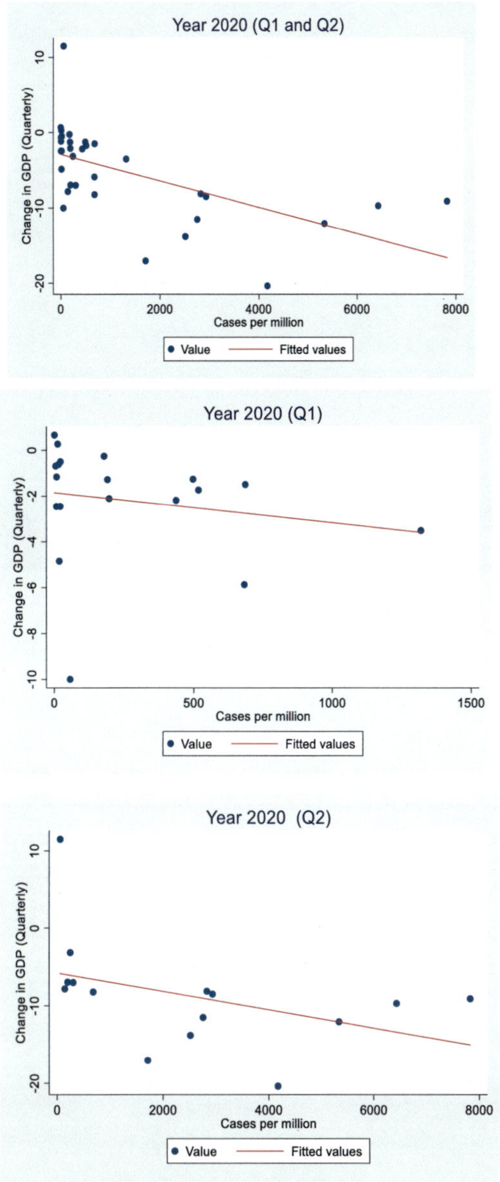

Fig. (1). COVID-19 Cases & Deaths and Change in GDP: We plot the number of COVID-19 deaths per million and the change in quarterly GDP for the first quarter of 2020 (Q1) and the second quarter of 2020 (Q2) in **Fig. 1a**, for Q1 in **Fig. 1b** and Q2 in **Fig. 1c**. We plot the number of COVID-19 cases per million and the change in quarterly GDP for Q1 and Q2 in **Fig. 1d**, for Q1 in **Fig. 1e** and Q2 in **Fig. 1f.**

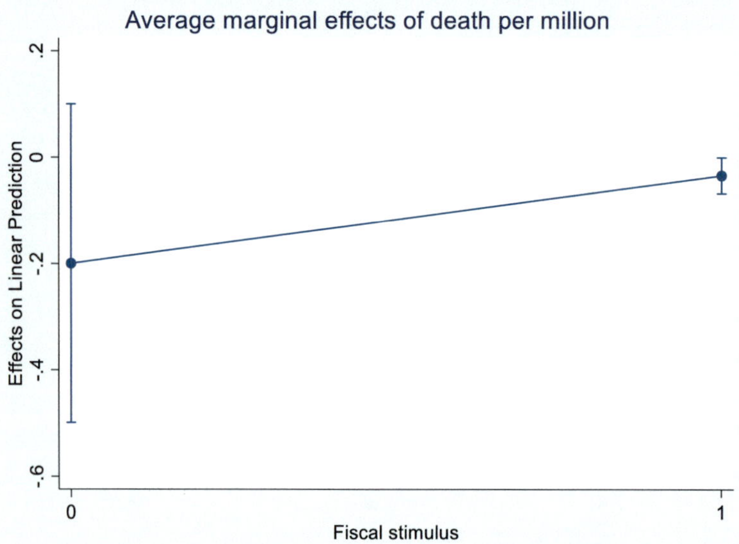

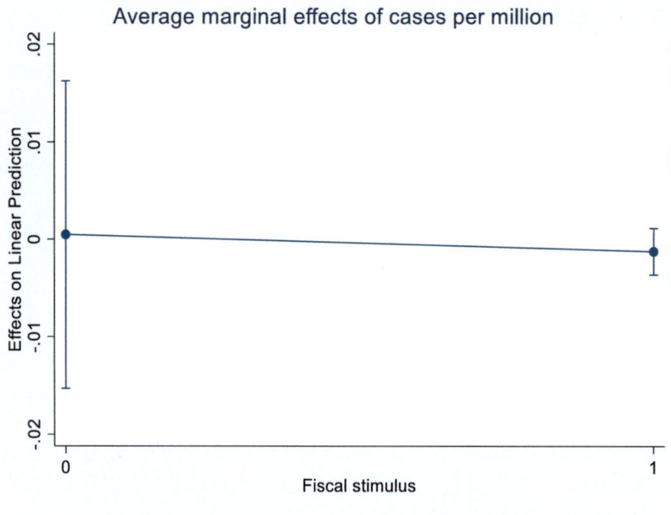

Fig. (2). Marginal effects of COVID19 on change in GDP – Impact of fiscal stimulus: In **Fig. 2a**, we plot the marginal effects of the number of COVID19 deaths per million on change in GDP, and in **Fig. 2b**, we plot marginal effects of the number of COVID19 cases on change in GDP. On the X-axis, 0 represents quarter 1, which is pre fiscal stimulus period and 1 represents quarter 2, which is post fiscal stimulus period.

In Table **2**, we provide regression results for equation (1), examining the impact of COVID deaths and infections on GDP. The negative and significant coefficient indicates an inverse relationship between death per million and GDP change and between infected cases per million and GDP change. We include country-fixed effects and report the results in column 3 for death per million and in column 4 for cases per million. We continue to find that an increase in the number of cases and deaths due to COVID-19 negatively affects GDP.

In columns (1) and (2), we regress the change in GDP on the number of COVID-related deaths per million and in columns (3) and (4), we regress the change in GDP on the number of COVID cases. In columns 2 and 4, we include the country-fixed effects. The sample size is 34 in each of the four regressions.

In Table **3**, we repeat our analysis of Table **2** with additional controls for cultural and institutional factors. The inclusion of these additional controls does not change our findings. We continue to observe a negative relationship between COVID-19-related death and infections and the change in GDP.

Table 2. Impact of COVID deaths and cases on GDP.

-	(1)	(2)	(3)	(4)
Death per million	-0.0201***	-0.0230***	-	-
-	(0.004)	(0.007)	-	-
Cases per million	-	-	-0.0018***	-0.0021***
-	-	-	(0.000)	(0.001)
Constant	-2.9400***	-4.8341	-2.8788***	-4.8065
-	(0.878)	(5.662)	(1.001)	(5.986)
Country FE	No	Yes	No	Yes
R-squared	0.452	0.619	0.345	0.574

Table 3. Impact of COVID deaths and cases on GDP: cultural and institutional controls.

-	(1)	(2)	(3)	(4)
Death per million	-0.0220***	-	-0.0228***	-
-	(0.006)	-	(0.007)	-
Cases per million	-	-0.0015**	-	-0.0021**
-	-	(0.001)	-	(0.001)
Power distance index (PDI)	0.0837	0.0166	-0.0170	0.0060
-	(0.104)	(0.115)	(0.999)	(1.076)
Individualism	0.0647	0.0109	0.0333	0.0032
-	(0.066)	(0.073)	(0.185)	(0.198)
Masculinity	-0.0301	-0.0131	0.0240	-0.0207
-	(0.054)	(0.062)	(0.123)	(0.133)

(Table 3) cont.....

-	(1)	(2)	(3)	(4)
Uncertainty avoidance index (UAI)	-0.0186	-0.0254	-0.0347	-0.0747
-	(0.055)	(0.064)	(0.254)	(0.275)
Long term orientation	0.0324	-0.0198	0.0672	0.0398
-	(0.058)	(0.064)	(0.163)	(0.174)
Indulgence *versus* restraint	-0.0448	-0.0878	0.0461	-0.0354
-	(0.087)	(0.098)	(0.186)	(0.196)
Government stability	-	-	-3.4655	-2.6950
-	-	-	(4.563)	(4.871)
Investment profile	-	-	-3.8256	-4.0990
-	-	-	(7.518)	(8.080)
Internal conflicts	-	-	2.6509	4.1893
-	-	-	(2.715)	(2.983)
Military in politics	-	-	-4.2324	-5.9935
-	-	-	(13.804)	(14.855)
Religious tensions	-	-	0.0534	1.7015
-	-	-	(3.042)	(3.300)
Law and order	-	-	4.0109	4.4205
-	-	-	(10.130)	(10.886)
Ethnic groups	-	-	-0.2924	0.1167
-	-	-	(6.595)	(7.102)
Democratic accountability	-	-	0.5749	1.8934
-	-	-	(2.863)	(3.127)
Constant	-7.4032	3.3144	28.8807	13.4455
-	(11.987)	(13.069)	(156.624)	(168.626)
-	-	-	-	-
Observations	28	28	28	28
R-squared	0.525	0.371	0.600	0.538

In columns (1) and (3), we regress the change in GDP on the number of COVID-related deaths per million and in columns (2) and (4), we regress the change in GDP on the number of COVID cases. Detailed variable definitions are provided in appendix C.

Next, in Table **4**, we examine the impact of government stimulus in moderating the effects of COVID-19 deaths and cases on GDP change. Stimulus by governments across the world is enacted in the last week of March or at the beginning of April (see Appendix A). The GDP is reported every quarter hence we use quarter 1 as the pre-stimulus period and quarter 2 as the post-stimulus period, *i.e.*, the fiscal stimulus dummy is zero for quarter 1 and is one for quarter 2. We find the interaction term for fiscal stimulus dummy & death per million and for fiscal stimulus dummy & cases per million to be insignificant, suggesting no change in the impact of COVID-19 cases and deaths on the real economy in the post-stimulus period.

Table 4. GDP and Stimulus.

-	(1)	(2)
Death per million	-0.1995	-
-	(0.138)	-
Fiscal stimulus dummy	-2.0021	-3.0594
-	(2.818)	(3.418)
Fiscal stimulus dummy * Death per million	0.1659	-
-	(0.125)	-
Cases per million	-	0.0005
-	-	(0.007)
Fiscal stimulus dummy * Cases per million	-	-0.0017
-	-	(0.007)
Constant	-4.7559	-4.8530
-	(5.508)	(6.168)
Country FE	Yes	Yes
R-squared	0.691	0.612
Standard errors in parentheses	-	-
*** p<0.01, ** p<0.05, * p<0.1	-	-

In columns (1), we regress the change in GDP on the number of COVID-related deaths per million, and in columns (2), we regress the change in GDP on the number of COVID cases. The fiscal stimulus dummy takes a value of zero for the first quarter and one for the second quarter. The sample size is 34 in each of the four regressions.

Impact of COVID on Stock Market: Moderating Effect of Fiscal Stimulus

In Table **5,** we provide descriptive statistics for our stock market analysis. We observe an average daily increase of 0.09 in the infection rate and 0.11 in the daily death rate during our sample period for the countries we study. Our infection rate and death rates are similar to Ashraf (2020), who reports a daily an infection rate of 0.18 and a daily death rate of 0.19 for a period from January 22 to April 17th 2020 [1]. Our sample though starts from the same date but is till 18th of August.

In (Fig. **3a**), we plot the scatter graph and trendline for the index return and rate of increase in death, and in (Fig. **3d**), we provide a similar plot for index return and rate of increase in the number of cases. The negative slope of the trendline indicates a decrease in index returns for the increase in the COVID-19 infection rate and death rate. In (Figs. **3b** and **3c**), we separately plot the graph in (Fig. **1a**) for stock market performance and the increase in death rate related to COVID-19 in pre-stimulus and post-stimulus periods, respectively. Similarly, in (Figs. **3e** and **3f**), we plot separate graphs for pre-stimulus and post-stimulus periods for the increase in infection rate. For the post-stimulus period, the slope becomes positive, indicating a positive effect of COVID-19 cases and deaths on stock market returns in the post-stimulus period.

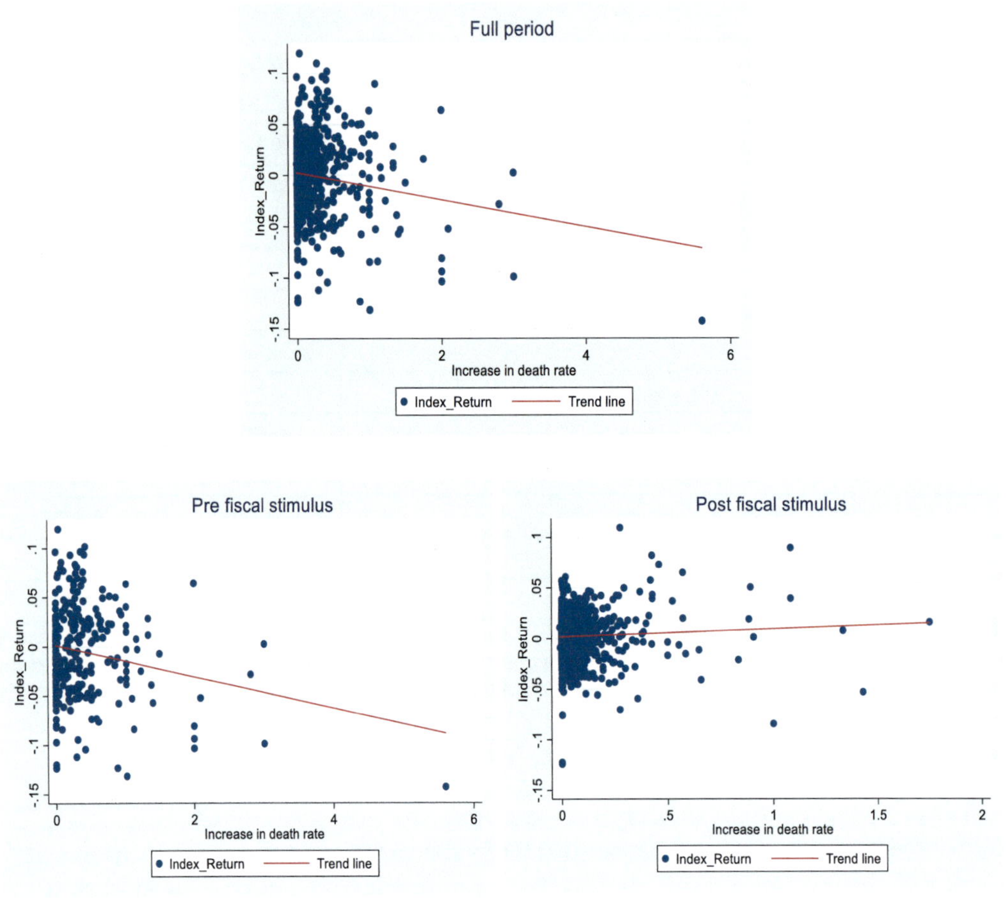

(Fig. 3) contd.....

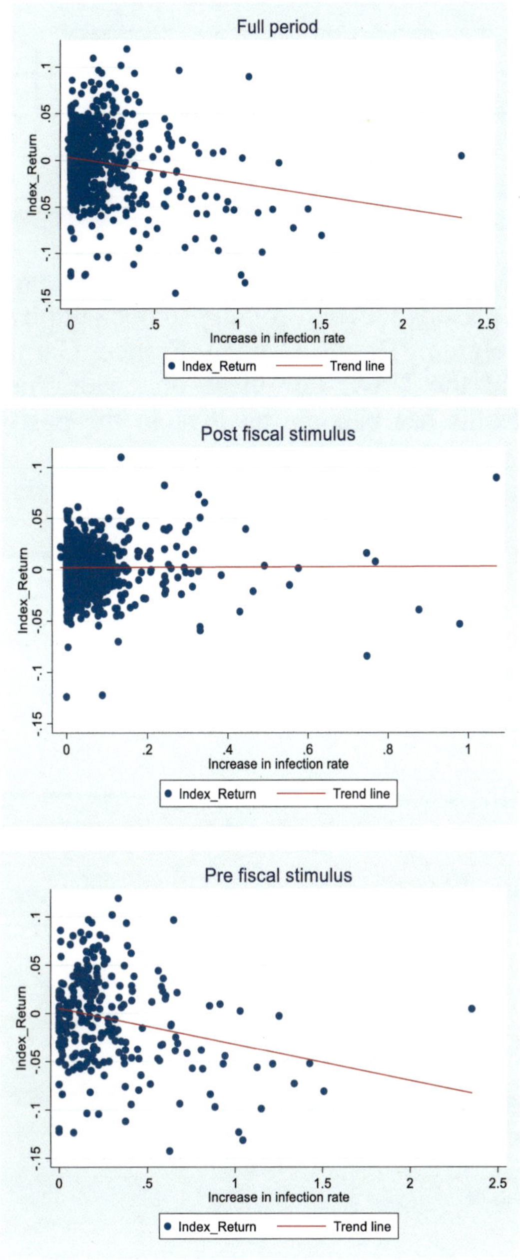

Fig. (3). COVID-19 cases & deaths and Stock market performance: We plot the increase in COVID-19 death rate and index returns for the overall sample **(Fig. 3a)**, for the pre-fiscal stimulus period (**Fig. 3b**) and post-stimulus period (**Fig. 3c**). We plot the increase in COVID-19 infection rate and index returns for the overall sample (**Fig. 3d**), for the pre-fiscal stimulus period (**Fig. 3e**), and the post-stimulus period (**Fig. 3f**).

Table 5. Descriptive statistics for stock market analysis (N=1959).

Variable	Mean	Std. Dev.	Min	Max
Increase in death rate	0.105	0.579	-0.010	22.611
Increase in infection rate	0.087	0.691	-0.015	29.663
Index_Return	0.001	0.025	-0.143	0.120

This table reports the summary statistics of variables used in our index returns analysis.

In (Fig. **4**), we plot the marginal effect of the death rate on stock markets in the pre and post-stimulus periods for each country in our sample. We observe positive slop for Australia, Belgium, Brazil, Canada, France, Germany, Japan, Mexico, Netherlands, UK, and the USA. For these countries, the marginal effect of COVID-19-related deaths has become positive in the post-stimulus period.

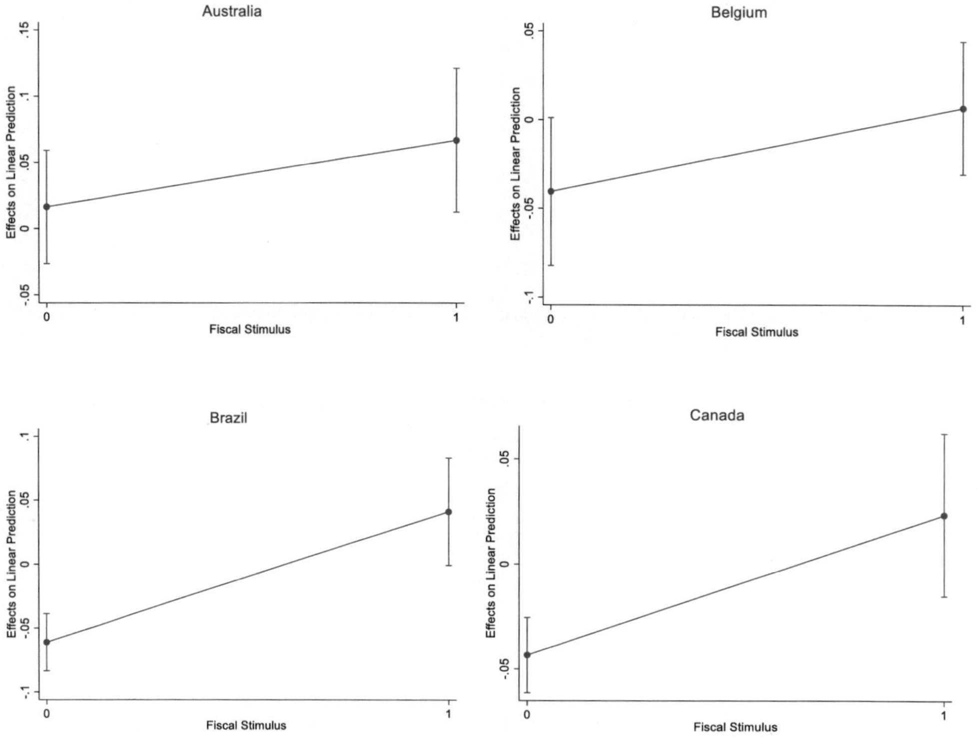

(Fig. 4) contd.....

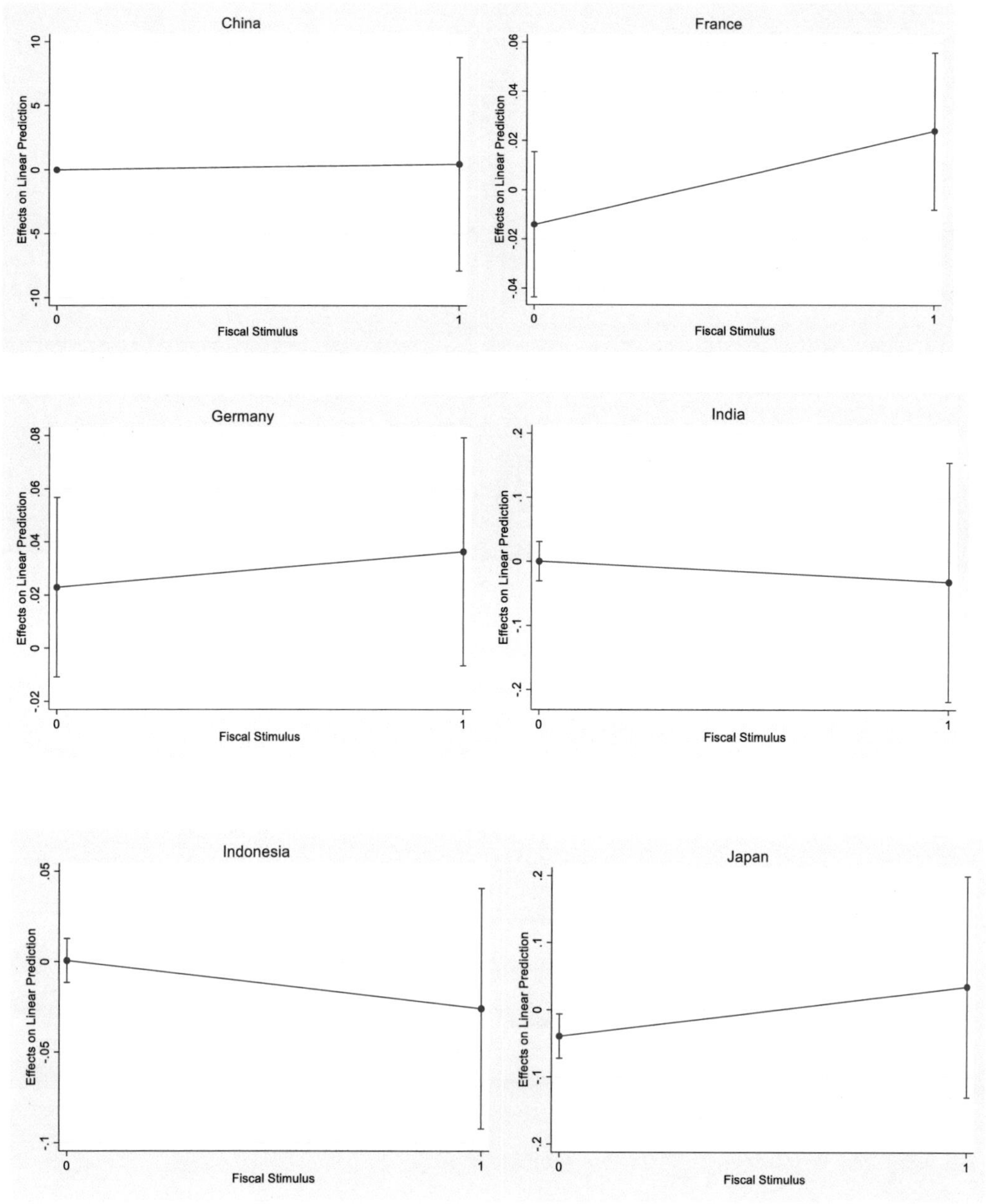
China
10
5
0
-5
-10
Effects on Linear Prediction
0
1
Fiscal Stimulus
France
.06
.04
.02
0
-.02
-.04
Effects on Linear Prediction
0
1
Fiscal Stimulus
Germany
.08
.06
.04
.02
0
-.02
Effects on Linear Prediction
0
1
Fiscal Stimulus
India
.2
.1
0
-.1
-.2
Effects on Linear Prediction
0
1
Fiscal Stimulus
Indonesia
.05
0
-.05
-.1
Effects on Linear Prediction
0
1
Fiscal Stimulus
Japan
.2
.1
0
-.1
-.2
Effects on Linear Prediction
0
1
Fiscal Stimulus

(Fig. 4) contd.....

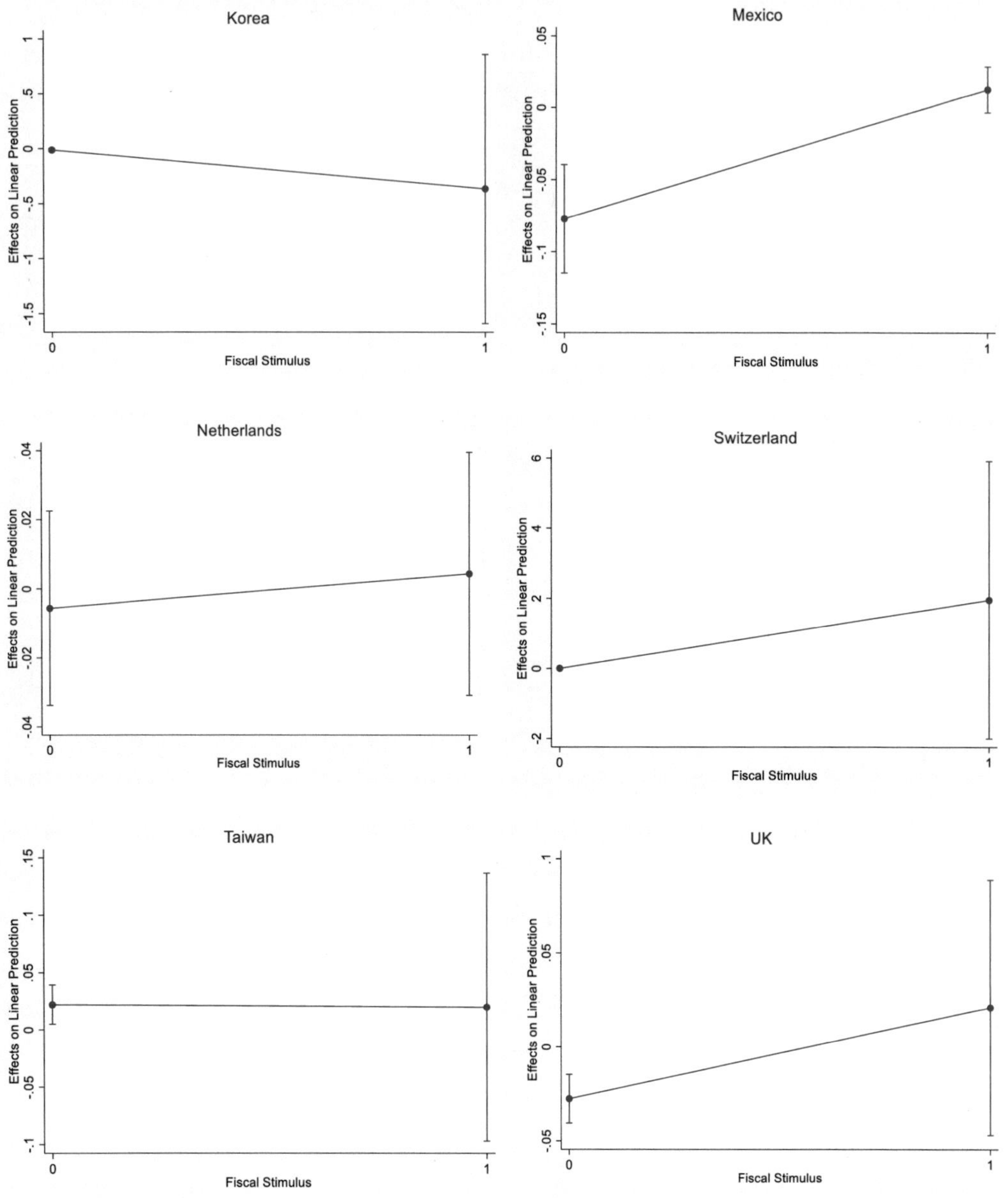
Korea
Effects on Linear Prediction
-1.5 -1 -.5 0 .5 1
0 1
Fiscal Stimulus
Mexico
Effects on Linear Prediction
-.15 -.1 -.05 0 .05
0 1
Fiscal Stimulus
Netherlands
Effects on Linear Prediction
-.04 -.02 0 .02 .04
0 1
Fiscal Stimulus
Switzerland
Effects on Linear Prediction
-2 0 2 4 6
0 1
Fiscal Stimulus
Taiwan
Effects on Linear Prediction
-.1 -.05 0 .05 .1 .15
0 1
Fiscal Stimulus
UK
Effects on Linear Prediction
-.05 0 .05 .1
0 1
Fiscal Stimulus

(Fig. 4) contd.....

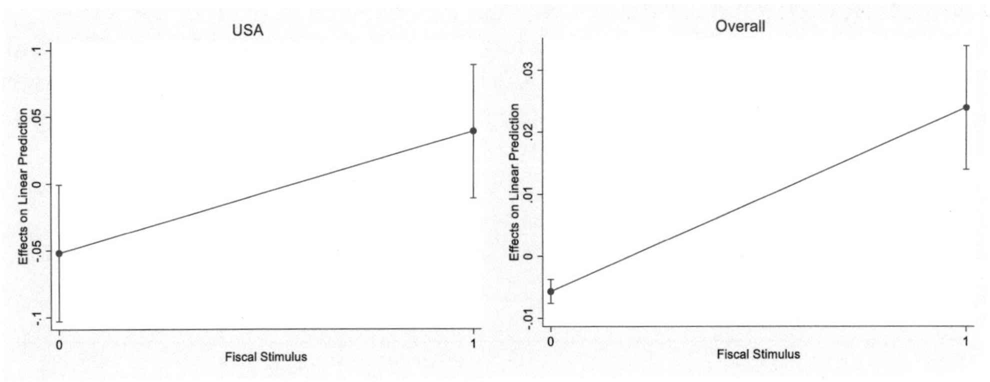

Fig. (4). Marginal effects of COVID-19 on stock market performance - Impact of fiscal stimulus (country-wise analysis).

In the following figures, we plot the marginal effects of COVID19 deaths on index return for each of our sample countries. On X-axis, 0 represents the pre-fiscal stimulus period, and 1 represents the post-fiscal stimulus period.

In Columns (1) and (2) of Table **6**, we report our multivariate regression results for index returns over the increase in death rates and increase in infection rate respectively. We find a negative and significant coefficient for both increase in death rate and an increase in infection rate, indicating an inverse relationship for COVID-19-related daily death rate as well as infection rate and index return. In column 3, we study the impact of fiscal stimulus, on the relationship between the death rate and index return. We include a dummy variable for the fiscal stimulus that takes a value of one for the post-stimulus period and zero otherwise. We also include an interaction term between the fiscal stimulus dummy and the increase in death rates to study the effect of COVID-related death rates on the stock index return in the post-stimulus period. We observe a positive and significant coefficient on the interaction term indicating a positive relationship between death rate and stock market performance in the post-stimulus period, *i.e.*, the higher the death rate due to COVID-19, the higher the stock return in the post-stimulus period. In column 4, we repeat a similar exercise to study the impact of an increase in infection rate on stock market return in the post-stimulus period. Our results indicate that stimulus moderates the relationship between infection rate and stock market returns. The higher the infection rate, the higher the stock market returns in the post-stimulus period.

In Table 7, we estimate the impact of death rate on index return in the post-stimulus period for each of the countries in our sample. The interaction term between fiscal stimulus dummy and increase in death rate is positive and significant for Belgium, Brazil, Canada, France, Mexico, and the USA. The interaction term is positive, albeit insignificant, for Australia, China, Germany, Japan, Netherlands, Switzerland and the UK. Overall, we find that the negative impact of the COVID death rate on the stock market has been mitigated by the fiscal stimulus provided by the majority of the countries in our sample.

Table 6. Impact of COVID deaths and number of cases on Index Returns.

-	(1)	(2)	(3)	(4)
Increase in death rate	-0.0057***	-0.0057***	-	-
-	(0.001)	(0.001)	-	-
Fiscal stimulus dummy	-	0.0068***	-	0.0079***
-	-	(0.001)	-	(0.001)
Fiscal stimulus dummy * Increase in death rate	-	0.0296***	-	-
-	-	(0.005)	-	-
Increase in infection rate	-	-	-0.0041***	-0.0037***
-	-	-	(0.001)	(0.001)
Fiscal stimulus dummy * Increase in infection rate	-	-	-	0.0215**
-	-	-	-	(0.009)
Constant	0.0002	-0.0068***	0.0002	-0.0075***
-	(0.002)	(0.003)	(0.002)	(0.003)
R-squared	0.021	0.051	0.016	0.036
Country FE	Yes	Yes	Yes	Yes
Standard errors in parentheses	-	-	-	-
*** p<0.01, ** p<0.05, * p<0.1	-	-	-	-

In Column (1), we regress the index return on the increase in COVID-related death rate, and in Column (2), we add the control for fiscal stimulus dummy and its interaction. In Column (3), we regress the index return on the increase in the COVID infection rate, and in Column (4), we add the control for the fiscal stimulus dummy and its interaction. Index returns are measured as the daily change in the stock index level of a country. An increase in the death rate is measured as the daily growth in the number of COVID-19 death. An increase in infection rate is measured as the daily growth in COVID-19 confirmed cases in a country. Fiscal stimulus is a dummy variable that takes a value of one for the post-stimulus announcement period and zeroes otherwise.

Table 7. Country-wise Multivariate analysis- Impact of COVID deaths and number of cases on Index Returns.

Variables	Australia	Belgium	Brazil	Canada	China	France	Germany	India	Indonesia
Increase in death rate	0.02	-0.04*	-0.06***	-0.04***	-0.00***	-0.01	0.02	0.00	0.00
-	(0.02)	(0.02)	(0.01)	(0.01)	(0.00)	(0.01)	(0.02)	(0.02)	(0.01)
Fiscal stimulus dummy	0.02***	-0.04**	-0.05***	-0.01	0.00	0.02**	0.03**	0.01	0.01
-	(0.01)	(0.01)	(0.01)	(0.01)	(0.00)	(0.01)	(0.01)	(0.01)	(0.01)
Fiscal stimulus dummy X Increase in death rate	0.05	0.05*	0.10***	0.07***	0.45	0.04*	0.01	-0.03	-0.03
	(0.03)	(0.03)	(0.02)	(0.02)	(4.22)	(0.02)	(0.03)	(0.10)	(0.03)
Constant	-0.02***	0.04***	0.05***	0.01*	0.00	-0.01**	-0.03**	-0.00	-0.01
-	(0.01)	(0.01)	(0.01)	(0.01)	(0.00)	(0.01)	(0.01)	(0.01)	(0.01)
Observations	110	99	105	109	136	118	108	108	98
R-squared	0.130	0.063	0.246	0.195	0.196	0.120	0.102	0.010	0.035
-	Israel	Japan	Korea	Mexico	Netherlands	Switzerland	Taiwan	UK	USA
Increase in death rate	0.03***	-0.04**	-0.01*	-0.08***	-0.01	0.00	0.02**	-0.03***	-0.05**
-	(0.01)	(0.02)	(0.01)	(0.02)	(0.01)	(0.01)	(0.01)	(0.01)	(0.03)
Fiscal stimulus dummy	-	-0.00	0.00	-0.04***	0.03**	0.01	0.01***	-0.01	-0.01
-	-	(0.00)	(0.00)	(0.01)	(0.02)	(0.01)	(0.00)	(0.01)	(0.01)
Fiscal stimulus dummy X Increase in death rate	-	0.07	-0.35	0.09***	0.01	1.95	-0.00	0.05	0.09**
-	-	(0.08)	(0.62)	(0.02)	(0.02)	(2.00)	(0.06)	(0.03)	(0.04)
Constant	-0.00	0.00	-0.00	0.04***	-0.03*	-0.01	-0.01***	0.01	0.01
-	(0.00)	(0.00)	(0.00)	(0.01)	(0.01)	(0.00)	(0.00)	(0.01)	(0.01)
Observations	57	123	123	102	103	112	124	110	114
R-squared	0.238	0.061	0.040	0.171	0.131	0.033	0.107	0.169	0.076

We regress the index return on the increase in COVID-related death rate along with the control for fiscal stimulus dummy and its interaction for each of the countries in our sample.

CONCLUSION

We study the impact of COVID-19 infections and deaths on the economic conditions and stock market performance for the 18 countries that yahoo finance provides information of. We find a negative and statistically significant impact of COVID-19-related infections and deaths on both the GDP as well as the stock index returns. The government of the countries in our sample provided fiscal stimulus to revive their economies and stock markets. We study if there are moderating effects of fiscal stimulus on the relationship between COVID-19 infections & deaths and the GDP & stock market performance. Our empirical analysis shows no relationship between COVID-19 cases and deaths and GDP in the post-stimulus periods. For the stock markets, we find an increase in index returns for the increase in COVID-19 cases and deaths in the post-stimulus period. The fiscal stimulus moderates the effects of COVID-19 on the GDP and the stock markets for the countries in our sample.

CONSENT FOR PUBLICATION

Not applicable.

CONFLICT OF INTEREST

The authors declare no conflict of interest, financial or otherwise.

ACKNOWLEDGEMENTS

Declared none.

REFERENCES

[1] Ashraf BN. Economic impact of government interventions during the COVID-19 pandemic: International evidence from financial markets. J Behav Exp Finance 2020; 27: 100371. [http://dx.doi.org/10.1016/j.jbef.2020.100371] [PMID: 32835011]

[2] Ashraf BN. Stock markets' reaction to COVID-19: Cases or fatalities? Res Int Bus Finance 2020; 54: 101249. [http://dx.doi.org/10.1016/j.ribaf.2020.101249] [PMID: 34170989]

[3] Erdem O. Freedom and stock market performance during Covid-19 outbreak. Finance Res Lett 2020; 36: 101671. [http://dx.doi.org/10.1016/j.frl.2020.101671] [PMID: 32837375]

[4] Zhang D, Hu M, Ji Q. Financial markets under the global pandemic of COVID-19. Finance Res Lett 2020; 36: 101528. [http://dx.doi.org/10.1016/j.frl.2020.101528] [PMID: 32837360]

[5] Haroon O, Rizvi SAR. COVID-19: Media coverage and financial markets behavior—A sectoral inquiry. J Behav Exp Finance 2020; 27: 100343. [http://dx.doi.org/10.1016/j.jbef.2020.100343] [PMID: 32427152]

[6] Mazur M, Dang M, Vega M. COVID-19 and the march 2020 stock market crash. Evidence from

S&P1500. Finance Res Lett 2021; 38: 101690. [http://dx.doi.org/10.1016/j.frl.2020.101690] [PMID: 32837377]

[7] Goodell JW. COVID-19 and finance: Agendas for future research. Finance Res Lett 2020; 35: 101512. [http://dx.doi.org/10.1016/j.frl.2020.101512] [PMID: 32562472]

[8] Hofstede G. Culture's Consequences: Comparing Values, Behaviors, Institutions, and Organizations Across Nations, 2001. 2nd ed., Thousand Oaks, CA: Sage 2001.

CHAPTER 5

Psychological Distress and Consequences of COVID-19 Pandemic on Different Groups

Saimah Khan[1,*] and **Arshi H. Khan**[2]

[1] *Department of Chemistry, Integral University, Lucknow-226026, Uttar Pradesh, India*

[2] *Department of Business, Management and Commerce, Integral University, Lucknow, India*

Abstract: The novel coronavirus 2019 (COVID-19) is extensively spreading all over the world, causing unprecedented hazards to mental health globally. The global pandemic of COVID-19 has been strongly impacting humanity and continues to influence all segments of the population since its origin. While dealing with such a public health crisis, past experiences have witnessed generalised public fear and anxieties due to uncertainty, causality and lack of public health preparedness. Therefore, it is important to acknowledge the detrimental effect of COVID-19 on the mental health of individuals of different age groups. This chapter aims to explore the impact of this unprecedented atmosphere on the mental health of the elderly, healthcare workers, children, adolescents and young people, pre-existing mental health conditions, post COVID-19 patients, women, homeless people and refugees. The chapter presents the direct and indirect psychological impact of COVID-19 on the genera at the individual, societal and public health levels. It will discuss at length some emerging concepts of the causal routes of mental disorders and suggest some strategies to prevent and promote mental health problems in individuals during this crisis. For the general population at large, just like physical effects, it is important to address the impact of COVID-19 on mental health effects as well. Various studies reported that mental problems such as anxiety, depression and fear of getting infected were common among people of all age groups who responded to COVID-19. The important lessons to be learned so far can help to devise individual mental health recommendations, as well as improved interventions and preventions of public health approaches.

Keywords: Anxiety, Adolescent, Children, Covid-19, Depression, Elderly, Healthcare Workers, Homeless, Impact, Mental Disorder, Pandemic, Pre-existing Mental Condition, Post-traumatic Stress Symptoms, Refugees, Stress.

* **Corresponding author Saimah Khan**: Department of Chemistry, Integral University, Lucknow-226026, Uttar Pradesh, India; E-mail: saimah@iul.ac.in

INTRODUCTION

The World Health Organization (WHO) on 11th March 2020 identified the Coronavirus disease 2019 (COVID-19) caused by the novel severe acute respiratory problem coronavirus-2(SARS-CoV-2) as a pandemic [1]. COVID-19 has created a worldwide crisis. Lockdowns, lack of known schemes for controlling this pandemic, loss of work and jobs, overflow of patients in hospitals, closure of educational institutions and more such disruptions have led to a vast impact on every aspect of human life across the globe.

These aspects include work culture, change in the pattern of education, fear of death, physical and mental health conditions, family gestures and relationships. Daily such effects were being discussed on news channels and social media, but issues related to the impact of COVID-19 on mental health were least discussed.

WHO, on 18th March 2020, published a report on the introduction of mental health and psychosocial considerations for humans, addressing the impact of this health emergency on the mental health of the population [2]. As compared to recent pandemics or medical emergencies, the COVID-19 outbreak is larger in scale; their consequence is unprecedented and thus, makes it more unpredictable. To control the outbreak, serious measures have to be taken on the mental health of the community [3, 4].

The pandemic made a big impact on the mental health of people in both positive and negative ways. The work-from-home culture during the lockdowns has given people an opportunity to spend more time with their family and relatives. This, in turn, upgraded the feeling of contentment and psychological well-being. But this was limited to a smaller fraction of the population.

A strong negative and adverse impact on mental health is on the larger population due to COVID-19. Due to this pandemic, locked-down were implemented in many countries for a longer period. Rise in insecurity in jobs, and economic hardship [5, 6], domestic conflict [7, 8], substance abuse [9], and media consumption [10, 11] are considered major factors affecting mental health. In this current pandemic, various studies [12 - 14] confirm the rise in the number of cases of stress, depressive symptoms, anxiety, sleep disorders and suicidal tendency. Often, patients of COVID-19 suffer from anxiety, depression and also post-traumatic stress disorder. Medical practitioners were in fear of getting infected and also facing stigma from their family members and community. Due to the overwhelming workload, healthcare workers suffer from overtiredness anxiety and insomnia. Patients with non-infectious chronic diseases like diabetes, cancer, *etc.*, were highest among the people who got anxiety, depression and distress. Similar was the situation for patients suspected of COVID-19 infection, people who were under isolation due to precaution from COVID-19, and doctors and nurses also were highest among the people who got anxiety, depression and distress.

Mental health issues, like depression, anxiety and panic, were also found to be common in the general population due to confusion about the end of the COVID-19 situation, a question regarding the treatment of the disease which is still not in sight. Recently quoted mental issues combined with the delay in treatment of serious chronic diseases lead to the exacerbation of common pathologies and have activated somatic symptoms [15 - 18]. Furthermore, photos and videos around the media and social networking media of stressed and ill patients, increasing death count, dead bodies, *etc*., and messages from the community that they are not able to meet and even see their close ones dying in hospitals have caused great social distress [19].

It is also noted that the frontline workers and COVID-19 patients faced noticeable challenges, while the challenges and issues faced by the general population were unnoticed and not even addressed. Many studies show that among the general population, there were mental health issues like psychological stress, depression, anxiety, stress, the loneliness, which have emerged progressively during the period of COVID-19. Isolation during the lockdown and quarantine triggered the increase in the number of suicide and suicide attempts, specifically among the youth, which was the main concern. Besides this, the strict quarantine measures were very much unfamiliar [20] and infringed on the freedom of the person [21, 22]. Uniting with this physiological problem, the economic crisis and unemployment influenced the stressors, such as the use of tobacco and drug, alcohol, potential addiction like gambling, and excessive use of mobile for gaming and surfing, and there was also an increase in the rate of sexual abuse and domestic violence [23, 24]. Taken together, there is an urgent call to generate awareness towards policies to assist people through this challenging time and public mental health.

In this chapter, we will discuss the impact and influence of COVID-19 on the mental well-being of the following categories.

- Healthcare workers (HCWs)
- People with previously known mental disorders
- People Infected with COVID-19
- Elderly Population
- Children, Adolescent and young people
- Women
- Refugees

• Homeless Population

The following graph shows the trends of cases and deaths in the United States.

Impact of COVID-19 on the Mental Health of Health Care Workers

The pandemic, *i.e.*, COVID-19, is now a prime global health threat and severely risks mental health across the globe. Healthcare workers (HCWs) are the most exposed group to COVID-19 and are certainly at very high risk [25]. As per the reports of Centres for Disease Control and Prevention (CDC) as of 2nd February 2022, there were in total of 900109 cases of COVID-19 and 3514 deceased among healthcare personnel across the globe (Figs. **1** and **2**) [26].

HCWs faced exhaustion, stigma, detachment from families, fear of being infected and infecting their beloved ones, and pain of losing co-workers and patient who were under a considerable amount of stress and anxiety during the pandemic of COVID-19 [27]. It is tough for HCWs to make a balance between duties and personal fear of getting infected with COVID-19, and it can often cause conflict and differences among them [28].

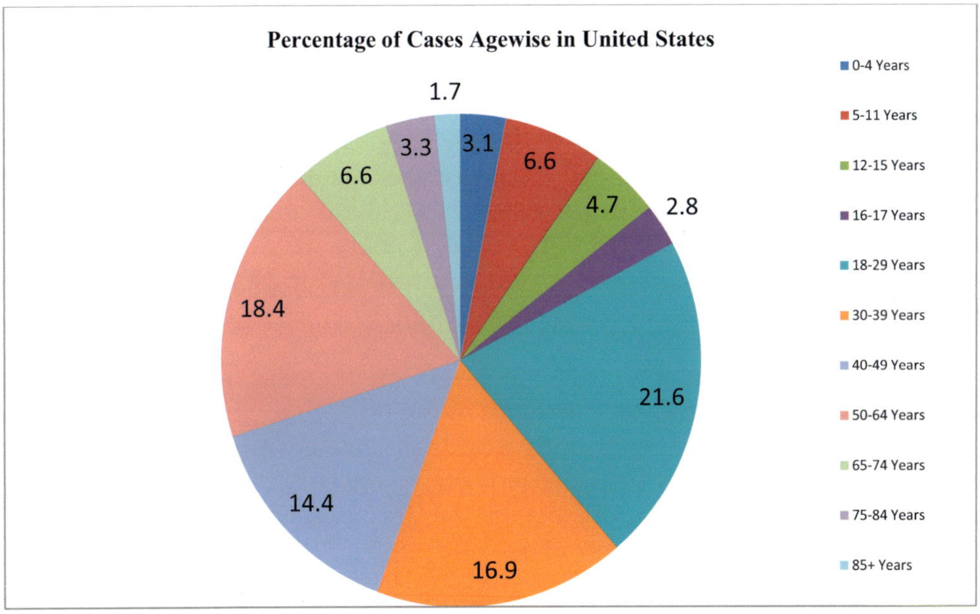

Fig. (1). Percentage of Cases Age-wise in the United States as reported on 2 Feb 2022 by the Centre of Disease Control and Preventions.

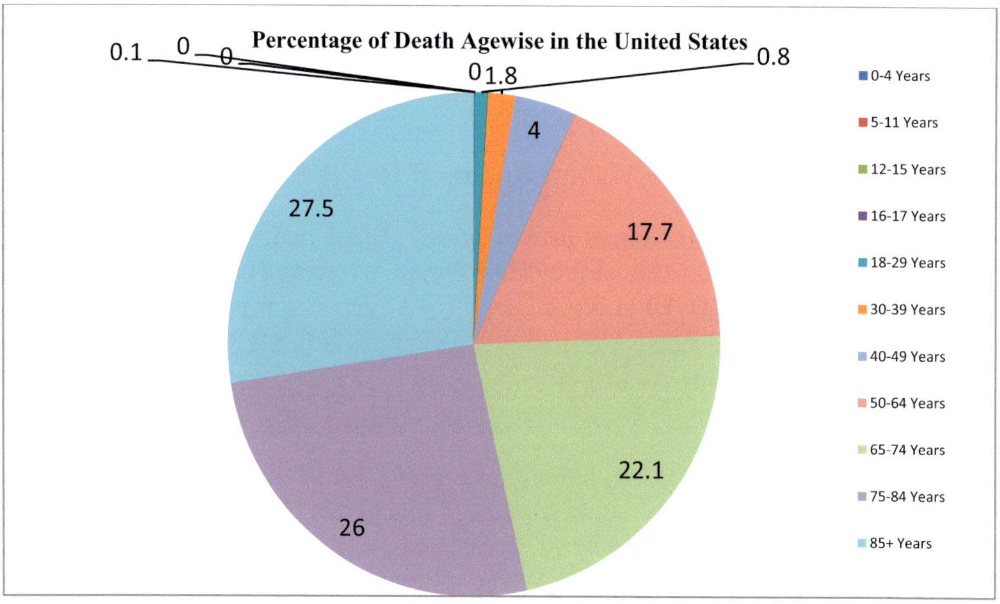

Fig. (2). Percentage of Deaths Age-wise in the United States as reported on 2 Feb 2022 by the Centre of Disease Control and Preventions.

Compared to doctors, nurses and medical staff are more susceptible to getting infected. Some other factors related to work that contribute to increased adverse psychological outcomes among HCWs is that apart from being employed on a part-time basis or having less experience, they are redeployed to look after affected patients and get increased exposure with covid positive patients. Other factors that contribute to increased risk are, isolation, either social or single, a team of workers having children at home, female gender, someone infected among members of a family, psychiatric disorders or physical problem, and further adversely affected HCWs mental health.

The outbreak of this major epidemic poses an increase in the demand for healthcare workers. The constant increase in the rate of cases, mortality, shortage of any specific medication, enormous workload, extensive media coverage, less availability of equipment for personal protection, and belief of insufficient support all factors contributed to excess mental burden among HCWs [29]. In such adverse circumstances still, it was expected from HCWs to do work for a longer time, while they were under extreme mental and physical load. When treating ill patients, they are at a higher risk of getting infected. Apart from this, similar to other persons, they are also exposed to a huge level of false and manipulated news which contribute to an increase in the level of anxiety [30]. Various studies reported that many HCWs got infected as they came in contact with infected patients of COVID-19 [31]. During the early phase of the COVID-19 epidemic, 29% of hospitalized patients were HCWs [32]. Through work in this scenario, there is the development of risk of various mental and psychological illnesses as well as emotional and physical distress in health care workers [29, 31].

The research conducted across the globe on various other infectious diseases, such as the Ebola virus, the Middle East Respiratory Syndrome (MERS), and severe acute respiratory syndrome (SARS), shows that a significant count of the study 1257 HCWs was assessed who have treatment of infected patients of SARS shows that in the initial stage dissemination of infection of the outbreak was fast, life-threatening, feeling of uncertainty, and significantly vulnerable indicated by cognitive and prevalence in somatic symptoms of anxiety [34]. On the other side, symptoms including anxiety, avoidance, traumatic stress, depression and burnout were reported even after the outbreak [33, 34]. Comparing the adverse psychological effects of SARS with COVID-19 found that the infected patients and deaths count in later have been much lesser than that of SARS [32]. A small section of people has been comparing the current scenario of the fast-spreading COVID-19 outbreak to "the end of the world". Hospitals were "overburdened," and there are many questions about the treatment of people's having pre-existing medical conditions [35]. The scenario of this COVID-19 all over the world potentially put HCWs and healthcare professionals in an unprecedented condition, forcing them to work under severe pressure [35, 36]. As result, healthcare workers are susceptible to experiencing mental and psychological problems. Thus, in this extremely unwanted situation, the mental health of HCWs and medical staff should be regarded as a crucial public health concern [32].

From the reports obtained from earlier global outbreaks and their psychosocial impacts on HCWs, an initial assessment of the mental health of HCWs and considering appropriate psychological empowerment is essential [37, 38]. Accordingly, significant practical and comprehensive measures to guard healthcare workers' mental health are essential [39]. Only a few studies are currently being focused on the psychological health of HCWs treating COVID-19 patients. Therefore, it is very important to study the articles which are addressed the status of HCWs' mental health during the COVID-19 outbreak. Further, various psychological interventions are given to improve the complete mental health of the healthcare workers (HCWs).

The study conducted on 1448 HCWs from nine Eastern Mediterranean Region (EMR) countries that responded to COVID-19, reported that 59.1% have anxiety, 57.5% have depression and 42.0% have stress. Examining the level of severity of patients, 26.6%, 19.2%, and 16.1% had extremely severe anxiety, depression and stress, respectively [40].

Another study in China among 123,768 healthcare workers reported that the prevalence of symptoms of anxiety and depression was 3.4% and 22.8%, respectively [41].

Another study on the effect of COVID-19 on the mental health of the Italian rehabilitation healthcare worker's cohort results suggested that the Italian HCWs showed an increased chance of suffering from anxiety, depression and stress during the COVID-19 outbreak [42].

The study consisted of 500 HCWs in Singapore to examine their anxiety, stress, psychological distress and depression, during the outbreak and to compare these parameters between medically trained and untrained health centre workers. From the results, it was reported that 68, *i.e.*, 14.5% individuals screened positive for anxiety, 42 *i.e.*, 8.9% for depression, 31 *i.e.* 6.6% for stress, and 36 *i.e.*, 7.7% for clinical concern of PTSD. Results also reveal that general anxiety was more among healthcare workers of a non-medical background rather than the medical background [43].

Outbreaks of the emerging COVID-19 pandemic, which occurred at regular intervals, have provoked an intense response from Health care workers (HCWs). During the pandemic, millions of HCWs keeping themselves on the front-line have to fight the disease. Concluding, it must be said that the prevalence of mental problems is significant among HCWs who responded to COVID-19 globally. Therefore, to initiate a fight for the mental well-being of HCWs who responded to COVID-19, special interventions need to be immediately implemented.

Impact of the COVID-19 Pandemic on the Mental Health of People with Previously known Mental Disorders

Patients with previously known mental health issues are highly susceptible to COVID-19 because this infection can aggravate mental health issues such as depression, anxiety, mental confusion, panic, psychosis and suicidal ideation.

The population with previously known psychiatric problems suggested exacerbating psychiatric symptoms [44]. According to a recent study that COVID-19 is showing a huge negative impact on patients with schizophrenia and other mental related problems [45], which may influence the well-being of these patients [46]. Therefore, it is possible to understand that this negative impact of COVID-19 will tend to lower the rate of recovery in patients with pre-existing mental problems.

Covid-19 infection and complications are higher in people with a pre-existing mental disorder as compared to people without a mental disorder, and this is because of comorbid conditions and cognitive deficiency [47]. Psychiatric sufferers are more likely to expose mildly to extreme worry about their physical health due to concerns that they'll have unknowingly reduced in size of the virus. They are also much less likely to apply powerful surviving strategies to control strain [48 - 50]. Similarly, other aspects are influencing the psychological health of patients, including delays in delivery of medicines, rise in financial trouble, shortage of getting admission to top care or outpatient clinics, stay at home for a longer period, and lack of basic resources make the living situations poor [51].

A recent study in Chile on patients with schizophrenia, and their caretakers revealed that COVID-19 infection tends to decrease the rate of recovery and mental well-being among these patients [52].

The study in Germany on 1522 patients with a previously known mental disorder reported that these individuals scored higher than healthy ones on all related scales (fear, anxiety and depression) of COVID-19. The rate of anxiety, depression and distress shows a significant impact on the patients with mental disorders, while the patients with somatic illness do not notably increase these parameters [53].

The study in the UK on 836 patients with a pre-existing mental health condition reported that these individuals were found to experience a higher rate of depression and suicidal ideation. It was also reported from the result that this individual shows a lower level score of well-being and a higher-level score of loneliness, defeat and entrapment [54].

Loss of sufficient resources in provider provision, worsening conditions in patients with mental disorders and hardships in providing support to mental health are also stated at some stage in the pandemic. During this time of unpredictability and difficulty related to survival, it is of utmost importance to provide support and guidance to these patients by providing proper management and care delivery systems.

Impact of the COVID-19 Pandemic on the Mental Health of People Infected with COVID-19

It is important to note that quarantine and isolation from relatives or loved ones help reduce infections, but on the other hand, it also reduces access to family, friends, and other social support systems that ultimately contribute to mental issues among the people infected with COVID-19. Furthermore, the recovered patients of COVID-19, recently discharged from the hospital, show high rates of post-traumatic stress symptoms (PTSS) [55]. Besides this, after discharge, patients in the intensive care unit (ICU) show the symptoms of post-intensive-care disorder accompanied by mental, cognitive and neurological ailment or dysexecutive syndrome [56]. According to a recently reported study that the risk of depression was higher in people who suffered from COVID-19 [57]. This is because the coronavirus has the ability to harm the brain by inducing massive cytokine activity in the brain [58]. Lastly, in the experiences with COVID-19 patients, it was reported that the rate of depression was higher in patients even after a year of recovery.

A cross-sectional study of 229 screened patients in Spain revealed that the COVID-19 survivors who were hospitalized only for the short term, exhibit a higher rate of psychiatric morbidity, neurocognitive disorder, and low quality of life [59].

Another study in Italy consisting of 402 adults surviving COVID-19 shows an increased rate of psychiatric sequelae, and a pathological score of a minimum of one disorder has been found in 55% of the sample taken. A higher rate of depression, anxiety and post-traumatic stress disorder (PTSD) is expected in most of the remnants. Furthermore, depression also increases the risk of all causes, leading to an increase in the mortality rate [60].

The study in China reported that depression and anxiety are significantly related to post-discharge residual symptoms, common among post covid patients who worry about recurrence and transferring of infection to others. Besides this, females were reported to be more susceptible to depression [61].

The study in Brazil reported that even after the acute stage of the disease, exposure of an individual to a large number of COVID-19 symptoms can increase the chances of anxiety, depression and post-traumatic symptoms [62].

The studies conclude that proper monitoring of post-Covid-19 patients should be done to prevent mental health problems. Some efforts toward public awareness to reduce stigma and discrimination may be warranted to reduce the secondary suffering related to the pandemic. Early interventions on coping methods of mental health education can benefit these people.

Impact of COVID-19 on the Elderly Mental Health

Pandemics have been known to cause significant social and psychological impacts. Uncertainty and misinformation that flow during pandemics give rise to mass hysteria and become a source of increased anxiety and fear, especially for the elderly. The elderly population is already at risk of catching infections because of their weak immune system and existing health conditions caused by ageing.

The remodelling of relationships puts the elderly at risk who are already prone to depression and anxiety, furthering the possibilities of "amplifying pre-existing conditions" [63].

Isolation often affects mental health. Many will develop stress, anxiety, and depression symptoms and will require external help. It is a concern that many of them will suffer in silence without communicating their distress, and there may not be any scope or resources in many parts of the world to assist or provide psychological support to such older people.

Older people are not always well versed with technology and have a problem with using smartphones. Therefore, it becomes imperative to explain to them in simpler terms the precautions to be followed during a pandemic. Various problems like meandering, irritability and psychotic symptoms, *etc*., and cognitive impairment can aggravate the panic, and taking care of simple hygiene measures could prove to be a difficult task. Elderly people with mental disorders, in the face of a crisis, are more prone to lurking risks of infection. Other reasons which led to their sub-standard care during the COVID-19 outbreak are the lack of proper healthcare utilization and discrimination against them. Older people sometimes become averse to social distancing and quarantine owing to the stress which is generated as a result of 'information overload. This paranoia and healthcare-related mistrust might lead to severe public health consequences.

Previous studies on infectious diseases have shown that there were more people mentally affected by pandemics than those who were physically infected by the disease, thus depicting the huge influence of the pandemics on the mental health of people [64].

According to a report (CDC- March 2020), more than 80% of death casualties belonged to the group aged above 65 years, thus indicating their higher vulnerability to the infection [65]. Reports from Korea have shown that 75.7 years was the average age of death, and the fatality rate of COVID-19 is directly proportional to age [66]. The incidences of severe infections increase with age, as shown by the following study. Incidents of severe infections were 19.8%, 43.2% and 81.3%, approximately in age groups 50-64, 65-79 and 80 years and above, respectively. The mortality rate of these age groups increased to 1.2%, 4.5%& 18.8% ($p = 0.025$), respectively [67].

According to a study conducted in China recently, there are negative effects of COVID-19 on the psychological health of individuals. A different study conducted on the general population depicted that 53.8% of the population reported being psychologically affected at a moderate to a severe level, 16.5% people reported symptoms of severe depression, 28.8% of respondents reporting symptoms of anxiety, and 8.1% reporting symptoms of stress [68]. During the pandemic, 37.1% of the elderly population experienced depression and anxiety [69].

Studies on elderly people have shown that social isolation is a "serious public health problem" that increases various risks of cardiovascular, autoimmune, and neurological problems, in addition to mental health problems.

Emotions like anger and fear should also be closely observed to understand the recent psychological effects caused by the COVID-19 pandemic. Fear becomes the main reason for various mental disorders when it is chronic or imbalanced, hence it requires greater attention.

There are several ways through which stress can be addressed. Remaining busy in healthy activities, setting up and adhering to a routine, routine physical exercise, yoga & meditation, relaxing activities, and spending time in activities that one enjoys are helpful strategies. Remaining in touch with family & friends with available means along with sharing and venting, can help. Limiting exposure to stressful information from media is important too. Identifying stress symptoms and taking early measures is the key. Sometimes it may be required for some people to seek help from professionals in the form of counselling, relaxation and supportive therapy.

Impact of COVID-19 on the Mental Health of Children, Adolescents and Young ones

The COVID-19 pandemic has affected the lives of people around the world. Even though children and adolescents are less in number for their positivity rate of the disease, the same cannot be true for their mental health. On 18th August 2020, due to this pandemic around 143 nations have shut down the schools and academic sectors globally, influencing the lives of 1,184,126,508 learners, comprising about 67.6% of students worldwide. Generally, it gives rise to huge stress levels in students, children and adolescents. Due to the lack of proper help and attention from qualified, trained teachers, these students are further facing distress, which will make their learning more costly for them and their families as they require extra time, support and assets. The academic and mental health of students can be adversely affected by this stress. The exposure of children to these incidents can exhibit the development of mental illnesses such as anxiety, depression, mood swings disorders, panic attacks, *etc.* [70]. Painful incidence stories along with separation from a circle of relatives and buddies, seeing or being privy to severely sick participants affected with coronavirus, or the loss of beloved ones or maybe considering themselves perhaps death from the virus would have a dangerous effect on the mental well-being of them. Due to COVID-19, some of the children also experience additional stress and drowsing issues, as their daily healthy routine has been disturbed. This pandemic may pose a risk of drug addiction among students, as they are uncertain about their future goals, academic and professional qualification and personal relation [71]. Children are additionally frightened, due to the fact they are scared not only about getting infected but also want their parents to work from home and not leave for work and go outside [72]. However, this pandemic is also uneven as some regions are not suffering from infection severely, while on the other side, numerous families have also lost their beloved ones. Similarly, in the COVID-19 setting, some youngsters have parents who are front-line workers, while others have parents who now do work from home or have these days been terminated [73]. In addition to this, school closure, campus closure and tour restrictions affected the academics of international college students globally. To reduce the spread of infection, many countries have restricted their borders to internationals creating problems for many college students as they do not have another place to stay. This unexpected closure of many countries to outsiders has positioned a big burden on college directors to make certain proper housing, sustenance, and safety of their global students. The new schooling platform web classes have helped both countrywide and worldwide college students to hold their schooling, while numerous children and college members are experiencing misery due to the fact they will not have the technological experience required to handle this new mode of communication. The COVID-19 pandemic has induced uncommon health and humanitarian disaster.

This is particularly correct when it comes to young individuals. The isolation, lack of contact with companions, and for many, the loss of emotional and financial security, influence their daily lives, including disturbance in their education. It leads to an increased risk of mental problems such as depression, tension, and sleep disorders in youth.

A meta-analysis of the consequences of COVID-19 on the mental health of children in Canada suggested that amid of COVID-19 pandemic, the mental health of children was negatively impacted [74].

A study in China consisting of 8140 school students (12–18 years old) reported that in middle and high school students, the percentage of depression and anxiety symptoms was found to be 43.7% and 37.4%, respectively. In China, it was also reported that the rate of depression was found to be higher in adolescents than in adults [75].

A study in the United States on the mental well-being of College Students amid COVID-19 reported that a higher level of anxiety and stress were common among

71% of students amid the COVID-19 outbreak. More than one stressor was also reported that increases the mental-related problems among students [76].

Again, in this third year of COVID-19, the negative impact of this infection on the mental health condition of kids and young people is continuously going on. According to the recent data provided by UNICEF, reported that the lockdowns harm every 1 in 7 children, while at the same time as more than 1.6 billion children have experienced the loss of education [77].

The general understanding of COVID-19 has elevated globally, yet its instantaneous and lengthy-term intellectual health impacts on children, adolescents and teenagers are hard to estimate. Important measures are taken to prevent the virus from spreading and handling this ambiguous condition may pose a threat to the mental well-being of the children. The initiative taken, such as school closure, restricting social interactions, implementing tour restrictions, closing sports activities, and switching all to online interaction system, causes emotional misery, fear, and anxiety amongst the children, adolescents and their caregivers. It is essential that the parents, and academic and health authorities defend and secure the mental health of children continuously *via* open conversation and promote professional counselling to cope with stressors. Special attention needs to be given to the children and youngsters, who are extra sensitive to the mental health disaster *via* a collaborative method employed along with their parents, educators, college administrators, counsellors and doctors.

Impact of COVID-19 on the Mental Health of Women

COVID-19 has changed the way things work for all segments of society. Nearly every segment of society is affected by stressors related to pandemics and women are no exception to this. Cases of domestic violence are known to intensify during a pandemic, worsening the already existing depression and anxiety disorders among women. Previous researches have shown that there are more self-reported cases of higher levels of stress, depression, anxiety and post-traumatic experiences in women.

In most parts of the world, women carry the responsibility of childcare and eldercare and as a result, mothers bear the load of parental stress. Parents are often involved in problems like financial crunch, social issues, unemployment, and alcohol abuse. These problems combined with the challenges of a pandemic have led to parents feeling more fearful, agitated, anxious and depressed. There is increased unpredictability and less control resulting from work-from-home and homeschooling children, all combined with limited outsourced help. These problems are more magnified in the case of single parents or parents having children with special needs.

According to a study conducted in Italy, among survey participants who wanted a child before the COVID-19 pandemic, 37% of them were reluctant to plan for a child after the outbreak of the pandemic [78]. This decrease was mainly due to the worries about the effects of the coronavirus on the pregnancy and the economic concerns. The delay caused by the pandemic in family planning of people was all the more stressful for women who were undergoing infertility treatments or for those women who were nearer to menopause.

Approximately one in seven perinatal women (this period includes the whole pregnancy and the year after delivery) have experienced enhanced levels of distress, anxiety and depression. For women who are experiencing a high-risk pregnancy, the percentage is even higher [79].

Pregnant women recruited after the onset of the pandemic were twice likely to report symptoms that indicated depression or anxiety disorder and substance use disorder [80]. In another study, it was found that 37.0% of participants endorsed elevated depressive symptoms (EPDS score 13 or above), 46.3% endorsed severely elevated anxiety, and 67.6% had clinically elevated pregnancy-related anxiety [81].

It is still unclear whether SARS-CoV-2 shows trans-placental transmission from infected pregnant women to their foetuses as the data are ambiguous [82] which further intensifies the pregnant women's stress.

Cases of domestic violence have been increasing at an alarming rate since the onset of the pandemic, according to the United Nations [83]. Calls to Intimate Partner Violence (IPV) emergency support lines have substantially increased in Spain, Italy and China during their respective lockdowns. Canada has documented a three times increase in call rates to Calls to Vancouver Battered Women's Support Services [84]. There has also been a 30% increase in similar calls in France and Brazil; the number is even higher. In China, shelter-in-places have reported a thrice increase in cases of domestic violence [85]. Latin America, where feticide rates are among the highest in the world, has seen a dramatic rise in reports of domestic violence [86].

A professional woman has to "Work from home" along with "Work for Home" for which there is very little appreciation and no monetary compensation. All these factors impact a devastating impact on such women's life resulting in the gradual deterioration of their physical and mental health, leading to stress, anxiety, burnout and depression.

Impact of COVID-19 on the Mental Health of Refugees

Disasters are often accompanied by an increase in depression, substance use disorder, posttraumatic stress disorder (PTSD), problems of child abuse and domestic violence in the general population. However, it is important to note that such disasters disproportionally affect vulnerable populations like the poor, patients with serious mental illness, and the at-risk immigrant and refugee populations.

Despite experiencing distress, immigrants and refugees are less to be referred to mental health services compared to the general population regardless of the COVID-19 pandemic. This may be due to cultural and linguistic barriers, or because of the stigma associated with seeking help for mental health. The lack of available translated information about COVID-19, and difficulties navigating the healthcare system leaves immigrants and refugees with limited English proficiency to the vast social media to obtain information and advice that may be inaccurate, stress-inducing, and even mythical [87].

Refugees and migrants are exposed extensively to various factors which may risk and negatively affect their mental health; such factors are difficult living conditions and living in neighbourhoods that are socially excluded and materially deprived. They are also not certain about their future and legal status, securing economic stability and enduring barriers to the labour market.

Outbreaks of pandemics such as COVID-19 generate fear and anxiety among people, leading to stigma towards particular groups of people, like people who have migrated legally or illegally. Soon after the outbreak of coronavirus, cases of stigmatization, racism and xenophobia were reported globally [88].

The sudden closure of market segments because of the pandemic in which labour and refugees work, such as cafes, food markets, hotels and restaurants or schools, leads to exacerbation of the prior existing stressful daily living conditions experienced by the socially vulnerable segment of the population.

The size of such a vulnerable segment of the population worldwide is surprising, it is almost 4% of the world population who lives outside their own country [89] and according to the reports of the United Nations High Commissioner for Refugees (UNHCR), 80 million people lives as refugees across the globe [90].

Studies have indicated that COVID-19 has deleteriously affected more on women's mental health conditions more in comparison to males. Many studies reported previously that women who migrated and are refugees of low-income countries were at risk for mental health issues [91].

Impact of COVID-19 on the Mental Health of Homeless People (HP)

A slice of the population that is particularly sensitive to psychological and health problems related to COVID-19 is certainly represented by the homeless people. Homeless individuals represent a silent minority in society, often not included in state censuses and with fewer opportunities for access to care services.

It is considered that 50% per cent of HP is suffering from some kind of mental disorder [92]. In Germany, from one meta-analysis [93] prevalence of 77.4% of HP, the population found Axis I disorders (Clinical disorders), 60.9% for drug addiction, and 55.4% population had addictive problems related to alcohol. The presence of these disorders increases the tendency of medical comorbidity, mortality due to suicide and risk of inability. Approximately 50% of the HP have issues of dual disorders, with a prevalence of 35% for mental disorders related to drug addiction.

Compared to the general population, homeless people are more likely to have previous psychopathological conditions or other chronic medical diseases, including bipolar personality disorder and schizophrenia.

Many people experiencing homelessness are engaged in high rates of substance abuse (including sharing of needles) due to chronic physical and mental conditions and often have less access to health care, all of which could lead to potential problems with quarantining, screening, and treating people who might have been affected with COVID-19. Personal Observation in search of symptoms of COVID-19 is lacking; same is the condition with access to diagnostic tests. Compliance with the isolation standards is impossible if the infection is confirmed.

Homeless people are also more likely to have a substance addiction than the general population. This leads to greater vulnerability to viral infections. The temporary closure of assistance services to homeless individuals with substance addiction probably represented an additional risk factor for possible relapses, with a consequent increase in mortality.

Limited knowledge of the mental health impact and issues related to the pandemic in this homeless section of the population is also a matter of concern, considering that these people are already suffering from vulnerable life, and the dangers and adverse conditions triggered the risk associated with the outbreak of this pandemic. Accordingly, these conditions increase the potential of their susceptibility to developing mental health problems.

CONCLUSION

From various reports, it is concluded that Covid-9 influences the mental health of the population in all age groups. The unprecedented risk caused by the COVID-19 pandemic may pose a risk to mental health in both developed and developing countries. To fight against this pandemic, mental well-being plays a crucial role. It is important to understand that fear due to the uncertainty of an infection caused by COVID-19 may be more dangerous than the virus itself. In this COVID-19 pandemic, mental problems are common among the people who are relatives of the sufferer, healthcare workers and other frontline workers. Generally, COVID-19 influences mental health in all age groups but shows a prominent negative impact on the mental health of susceptible groups such as pre-existing mental disorders, old-age people, younger ones and poor illiterate people. Therefore, it is crucial to develop policies that work to reduce the consequences of this pandemic. The policies must provide clear instructions, proactive protocols and effective communication pathways to alleviate the consequences of the pandemic. It is also reported that the interventions induced by COVID-19 to counterbalance the financial, social and role disturbance among the elderly, pre-existing mental conditions and homeless people are likely to significantly impact their mental health. Therefore, there is an urgent need for government policy that works on preventive measures for mental health problems of the general population.

CONSENT FOR PUBLICATION

Not applicable.

CONFLICT OF INTEREST

The authors declare no conflict of interest, financial or otherwise.

ACKNOWLEDGEMENTS

Declared none.

REFERENCES

[1] Euro.who.int/en [homepage on internet], World Health Organisation (WHO): WHO announces COVID-19 outbreak a pandemic.[updated on 12 Mar 2020]. Available from: https://www.euro.who.int/en/health-topics/health-emergencies/coronavir-s-covid-19/news/news/2020/3/who-announces-covid-19-outbreak-a-pandemic

[2] Who.int/doc [homepage on internet], WHO. Mental health and psychosocial considerations during the COVID-19 outbreak. [updated on 18 March 2020]. Available from: https://www.who.int/docs/default-source/coronaviruse/mental-health-considerations.pdf

[3] Pfefferbaum B, North CS. Mental health and the COVID-19 pandemic. N Engl J Med 2020; 383(6): 510-2.
[http://dx.doi.org/10.1056/NEJMp2008017] [PMID: 32283003]

[4] Holmes EA, O'Connor RC, Perry VH, *et al.* Multidisciplinary research priorities for the COVID-19 pandemic: a call for action for mental health science. Lancet Psychiatry 2020; 7(6): 547-60. [http://dx.doi.org/10.1016/S2215-0366(20)30168-1] [PMID: 32304649]

[5] Uutela A. Economic crisis and mental health. Curr Opin Psychiatry 2010; 23(2): 127-30. [http://dx.doi.org/10.1097/YCO.0b013e328336657d] [PMID: 20087188]

[6] Evans-Lacko S, Knapp M, McCrone P, Thornicroft G, Mojtabai R. The mental health consequences of the recession: economic hardship and employment of people with mental health problems in 27 European countries. PLoS One 2013; 8(7): e69792. [http://dx.doi.org/10.1371/journal.pone.0069792] [PMID: 23922801]

[7] Usher K, Bhullar N, Durkin J, Gyamfi N, Jackson D. Family violence and COVID-19: Increased vulnerability and reduced options for support. Int J Ment Health Nurs 2020; 29(4): 549-52. [http://dx.doi.org/10.1111/inm.12735] [PMID: 32314526]

[8] Mazza M, Marano G, Lai C, Janiri L, Sani G. Danger in danger: Interpersonal violence during COVID-19 quarantine. Psychiatry Res 2020; 289: 113046. [http://dx.doi.org/10.1016/j.psychres.2020.113046] [PMID: 32387794]

[9] Volkow ND. Volkow. ND. Collision of the COVID-19 and addiction epidemics. Ann Intern Med 2020; 173(1): 61-2. [http://dx.doi.org/10.7326/M20-1212] [PMID: 32240293]

[10] Gao J, Zheng P, Jia Y, *et al.* Mental health problems and social media exposure during COVID-19 outbreak. PLoS One 2020; 15(4): e0231924. [http://dx.doi.org/10.1371/journal.pone.0231924] [PMID: 32298385]

[11] Garfin DR, Silver RC, Holman EA. The novel coronavirus (COVID-2019) outbreak: Amplification of public health consequences by media exposure. Health Psychol 2020; 39(5): 355-7. [http://dx.doi.org/10.1037/hea0000875] [PMID: 32202824]

[12] Wang C, Pan R, Wan X, *et al.* A longitudinal study on the mental health of general population during the COVID-19 epidemic in China. Brain Behav Immun 2020; 87: 40-8. [http://dx.doi.org/10.1016/j.bbi.2020.04.028] [PMID: 32298802]

[13] Wang J, Alsop DC, Song HK, *et al.* Arterial transit time imaging with flow encoding arterial spin tagging (FEAST). Magn Reson Med 2003; 50(3): 599-607. [http://dx.doi.org/10.1002/mrm.10559] [PMID: 12939768]

[14] Plomecka MB, Gobbi S, Neckels R, *et al.* Mental health impact of COVID-19: a global study of risk and resilience factors. PsyArXiv 2020. [http://dx.doi.org/10.31234/osf.io/zj6b4]

[15] Tsamakis K, Triantafyllis A, Tsiptsios D, *et al.* COVID-19 related stress exacerbates common physical and mental pathologies and affects treatment (Review). Exp Ther Med 2020; 20(1): 159-62. [http://dx.doi.org/10.3892/etm.2020.8671] [PMID: 32509006]

[16] Giannitsi S, Tsinivizov P, Poulimenos LE, *et al.* [Case Report] Stress induced (Takotsubo) cardiomyopathy triggered by the COVID-19 pandemic. Exp Ther Med 2020; 20(3): 2812-4. [PMID: 32765776]

[17] Tsamakis K, Gavriatopoulou M, Schizas D, *et al.* Oncology during the COVID-19 pandemic: challenges, dilemmas and the psychosocial impact on cancer patients (Review). Oncol Lett 2020; 20(1): 441-7. [http://dx.doi.org/10.3892/ol.2020.11599] [PMID: 32565968]

[18] https://unsdg.un.org/resources/policy-brief-covid-19-and-need-action-mental-health

[19] Moris D, Schizas D. Lockdown During COVID-19: The Greek Success. *In Vivo* 2020; 34(3 suppl) (Suppl.): 1695-9. [http://dx.doi.org/10.21873/invivo.11963] [PMID: 32503831]

[20] Pfefferbaum B, North CS. Mental health and the Covid-19 pandemic. N Engl J Med 2020; 383: 510-2.

[21] Brooks SK, Webster RK, Smith LE, *et al.* The psychological impact of quarantine and how to reduce it: rapid review of the evidence. Lancet 2020; 395(10227): 912-20. [http://dx.doi.org/10.1016/S0140-6736(20)30460-8] [PMID: 32112714]

[22] The Lancet Infectious Diseases. The intersection of COVID-19 and mental health. Lancet Infect Dis 2020; 20(1217): 2020. [http://dx.doi.org/10.1016/S1473-3099(20)30797-0]

[23] Gautam. M, Thakrar. A, Akinyemi. E, Mahr. Current and future challenges in the delivery of mental health care during COVID-19. SN Compr Clin Med 2020. 2(7): 865–870. [http://dx.doi.org/10.1007/s42399-020-00348-3]

[24] Moris. D, Tsilimigras. DI, Schizas. D. Cancer and COVID-19. Lancet 2020; 396(10257): 1066.

[25] Alrubaiee GG, Al-Qalah TAH, Al-Aawar MSA. Knowledge, attitudes, anxiety, and preventive behaviours towards COVID-19 among health care providers in Yemen: an online cross-sectional survey. BMC Public Health 2020; 20(1): 1541. [http://dx.doi.org/10.1186/s12889-020-09644-y] [PMID: 33050896]

[26] CDC. Cases & Deaths among Healthcare Personnel. [Updated on 2 Feb 2022]. Available from: https://covid.cdc.gov/covid-data-tracker/#health-care-personnel

[27] Regly. E. Italian doctors' fatalities reach tragic levels as they fight COVID-19 in overburdened hospitals. The Globe and Mail 2020. Available from: https://www.theglobeandmail.com/world/article-italian-doctors-fatalities-reach-tragic-levels-as-they-fight-covid-1/

[28] Ho CS. Chee. CY, Ho. RC. Mental Health Strategies to Combat the Psychological Impact of COVID-19 Beyond Paranoia and Panic. Ann Acad Med Singap 2020; 49(3): 155-60. [http://dx.doi.org/10.47102/annals-acadmedsg.202043] [PMID: 32200399]

[29] Lai J, Ma S, Wang Y, *et al.* Factors associated with mental health outcomes among health care workers exposed to coronavirus disease 2019. JAMA Netw Open 2020; 3(3): e203976. [http://dx.doi.org/10.1001/jamanetworkopen.2020.3976] [PMID: 32202646]

[30] Schwartz J, King CC, Yen MY. King. C-C, Yen. M-Y. Protecting healthcare workers during the coronavirus disease 2019 (COVID-19) outbreak: lessons from Taiwan's severe acute respiratory syndrome response. Clin Infect Dis 2020; 71(15): 858-60. [http://dx.doi.org/10.1093/cid/ciaa255] [PMID: 32166318]

[31] Xiao H, Zhang Y, Kong D, Li S, Yang N. The Effects of Social Support on Sleep Quality of Medical Staff Treating Patients with Coronavirus Disease 2019 (COVID-19) in January and February 2020 in China. Med Sci Monit 2020; 26: e923549. [http://dx.doi.org/10.12659/MSM.923549] [PMID: 32132521]

[32] Zhu Z, Xu S, Wang H, *et al.* COVID-19 in Wuhan: Immediate Psychological Impact on 5062 Health Workers. medRxiv 2020; 100443. [http://dx.doi.org/10.1101/2020.02.20.20025338]

[33] Lee SM, Kang WS, Cho AR, Kim T, Park JK. Psychological impact of the 2015 MERS outbreak on hospital workers and quarantined hemodialysis patients. Compr Psychiatry 2018; 87: 123-7. [http://dx.doi.org/10.1016/j.comppsych.2018.10.003] [PMID: 30343247]

[34] Chong. M-Y, Wang. W-C, Hsieh. W-C. *et al.* Psychological impact of severe acute respiratory syndrome on health workers in a tertiary hospital. Br J Psychiatry 2004; 185(2): 127-33. [http://dx.doi.org/10.1192/bjp.185.2.127]

[35] Lima CKT, Carvalho PMM, Lima IAAS, *et al.* The emotional impact of Coronavirus 2019-nCoV (new Coronavirus disease). Psychiatry Res 2020; 287: 112915. [http://dx.doi.org/10.1016/j.psychres.2020.112915] [PMID: 32199182]

[36] Greenberg N, Docherty M, Gnanapragasam S, Wessely S. Managing mental health challenges faced

by healthcare workers during COVID-19 pandemic. BMJ 2020; 368: m1211. [http://dx.doi.org/10.1136/bmj.m1211] [PMID: 32217624]

[37] Li Z, Ge J, Yang M, *et al.* Vicarious traumatization in the general public, members, and non-members of medical teams aiding in COVID-19 control. Brain Behav Immun 2020; 88: 916-9. [http://dx.doi.org/10.1016/j.bbi.2020.03.007] [PMID: 32169498]

[38] Xiang YT, Yang Y, Li W, *et al.* Timely mental health care for the 2019 novel coronavirus outbreak is urgently needed. Lancet Psychiatry 2020; 7(3): 228-9. [http://dx.doi.org/10.1016/S2215-0366(20)30046-8] [PMID: 32032543]

[39] Kang L, Ma S, Chen M, *et al.* Impact on mental health and perceptions of psychological care among medical and nursing staff in Wuhan during the 2019 novel coronavirus disease outbreak: A cross-sectional study. Brain Behav Immun 2020; 87: 11-7. [http://dx.doi.org/10.1016/j.bbi.2020.03.028] [PMID: 32240764]

[40] Ghaleb Y, Lami F, Al Nsour M, *et al.* Mental health impacts of COVID-19 on healthcare workers in the Eastern Mediterranean Region: a multi-country study. J Public Health (Oxf) 2021; 43 (Suppl. 3): iii34-42. [http://dx.doi.org/10.1093/pubmed/fdab321] [PMID: 34642765]

[41] Zhang XR, Huang QM, Wang XM, *et al.* Prevalence of anxiety and depression symptoms, and association with epidemic-related factors during the epidemic period of COVID-19 among 123,768 workers in China: A large cross-sectional study. J Affect Disord 2020; 277: 495-502. [http://dx.doi.org/10.1016/j.jad.2020.08.041] [PMID: 32882506]

[42] Farì G, Sire A, Giorgio V, *et al.* Impact of COVID-19 on the mental health in a cohort of Italian rehabilitation healthcare workers. J Med Virol 2022; 94(1): 110-8. [http://dx.doi.org/10.1002/jmv.27272] [PMID: 34387886]

[43] Tan BYQ, Chew NWS, Lee GKH, *et al.* Psychological Impact of the COVID-19 Pandemic on Health Care Workers in Singapore. Ann Intern Med 2020; 173(4): 317-20. [http://dx.doi.org/10.7326/M20-1083] [PMID: 32251513]

[44] Vindegaard N, Benros ME. COVID-19 pandemic and mental health consequences: Systematic review of the current evidence. Brain Behav Immun 2020; 89: 531-42. [http://dx.doi.org/10.1016/j.bbi.2020.05.048] [PMID: 32485289]

[45] Kozloff N, Mulsant BH, Stergiopoulos V, Voineskos AN. Kozloff. N, Mulsant. B.H, Stergiopoulos. V and Voineskos. A N. The COVID-19 global pandemic: implications for people with schizophrenia and related disorders. Schizophr Bull 2020; 46(4): 752-7. [http://dx.doi.org/10.1093/schbul/sbaa051]

[46] Burrai J, Roma P, Barchielli B, *et al.* Psychological and emotional impact of patients living in psychiatric treatment communities during COVID-19 lockdown in Italy. J Clin Med 2020; 9(11): 3787. [http://dx.doi.org/10.3390/jcm9113787] [PMID: 33238610]

[47] Shinn. A K, Viron. M. Perspectives on the COVID-19 pandemic and individuals with serious mental illness. J Clin Psychiatry 2020; 81: 20com13412. [http://dx.doi.org/10.4088/JCP.20com13412]

[48] Chua SE, Cheung V, McAlonan GM, *et al.* Stress and psychological impact on SARS patients during the outbreak. Can J Psychiatry 2004; 49(6): 385-90. [http://dx.doi.org/10.1177/070674370404900607] [PMID: 15283533]

[49] Phillips LJ, Francey SM, Edwards J, McMurray N. Strategies used by psychotic individuals to cope with life stress and symptoms of illness: a systematic review. Anxiety Stress Coping 2009; 22(4): 371-410. [http://dx.doi.org/10.1080/10615800902811065] [PMID: 19333796]

[50] Solé B, Verdolini N, Amoretti S, *et al.* Effects of the COVID-19 pandemic and lockdown in Spain:

comparison between community controls and patients with a psychiatric disorder. Preliminary results from the BRIS-MHC STUDY. J Affect Disord 2021; 281: 13-23. [http://dx.doi.org/10.1016/j.jad.2020.11.099] [PMID: 33279864]

[51] Hao F, Tan W, Jiang L, *et al.* Do psychiatric patients experience more psychiatric symptoms during COVID-19 pandemic and lockdown? A case-control study with service and research implications for immunopsychiatry. Brain Behav Immun 2020; 87: 100-6. [http://dx.doi.org/10.1016/j.bbi.2020.04.069] [PMID: 32353518]

[52] Caqueo-Urízar A, Urzúa A, Ponce-Correa F, Ferrer R. Psychosocial Effects of the COVID-19 Pandemic on Patients With Schizophrenia and Their Caregivers. Front Psychol 2021; 12: 729793. [http://dx.doi.org/10.3389/fpsyg.2021.729793] [PMID: 34803806]

[53] Skoda EM, Bäuerle A, Schweda A, *et al.* Severely increased generalized anxiety, but not COVID-1--related fear in individuals with mental illnesses: A population based cross-sectional study in Germany. Int J Soc Psychiatry 2021; 67(5): 550-8. [http://dx.doi.org/10.1177/0020764020960773] [PMID: 33040668]

[54] O'Connor RC, Wetherall K, Cleare S, *et al.* Mental health and well-being during the COVID-19 pandemic: longitudinal analyses of adults in the UK COVID-19 Mental Health & Wellbeing study. Br J Psychiatry 2021; 218(6): 326-33. [http://dx.doi.org/10.1192/bjp.2020.212] [PMID: 33081860]

[55] Bo HX, Li W, Yang Y, *et al.* Posttraumatic stress symptoms and attitude toward crisis mental health services among clinically stable patients with COVID-19 in China. Psychol Med 2021; 51(6): 1052-3. [http://dx.doi.org/10.1017/S0033291720000999] [PMID: 32216863]

[56] Helms J, Kremer S, Merdji H, *et al.* Neurologic features in severe SARS-CoV-2 infection. N Engl J Med 2020; 382(23): 2268-70. [http://dx.doi.org/10.1056/NEJMc2008597] [PMID: 32294339]

[57] Zhang J, Lu H, Zeng H, *et al.* The differential psychological distress of populations affected by the COVID-19 pandemic. Brain Behav Immun 2020; 87: 49-50. [http://dx.doi.org/10.1016/j.bbi.2020.04.031] [PMID: 32304883]

[58] Rogers JP, Chesney E, Oliver D, *et al.* Psychiatric and neuropsychiatric presentations associated with severe coronavirus infections: a systematic review and meta-analysis with comparison to the COVID-19 pandemic. Lancet Psychiatry 2020; 7(7): 611-27. [http://dx.doi.org/10.1016/S2215-0366(20)30203-0] [PMID: 32437679]

[59] Mendez R, Balanza-Martinez V, Luperdi SC, *et al.* Short-term neuropsychiatric outcomes and quality of Life in COVID-19 survivors. medRxiv 2020. [http://dx.doi.org/10.1101/2020.09.23.20190090]

[60] Mazza MG, De Lorenzo R, Conte C, *et al.* Anxiety and depression in COVID-19 survivors: Role of inflammatory and clinical predictors. Brain Behav Immun 2020; 89: 594-600. [http://dx.doi.org/10.1016/j.bbi.2020.07.037] [PMID: 32738287]

[61] Wu C, Hu X, Song J, *et al.* Mental health status and related influencing factors of COVID-19 survivors in Wuhan, China. Clin Transl Med 2020; 10(2): e52. [http://dx.doi.org/10.1002/ctm2.52] [PMID: 32508037]

[62] Ismael F, Bizario JC, Battagin T, *et al.* Post-infection depression, anxiety and PTSD: a retrospective cohort study with mild COVID-19 patients. Prog Neuropsychopharmacol Biol Psychiatry 2021; 111: 110341. [http://dx.doi.org/10.1016/j.pnpbp.2021.110341] [PMID: 33940097]

[63] Ho CSH, Chee CYI, Ho RCM. Mental health strategies to combat the psychological impact of coronavirus disease 2019 (COVID-19) Beyond paranoia and panic. Ann Acad Med Singap 2020; 49(3): 155-60. [http://dx.doi.org/10.47102/annals-acadmedsg.202043] [PMID: 32200399]

[64] Reardon S. Ebola's mental-health wounds linger in Africa. Nature 2015; 519(7541): 13-4. [http://dx.doi.org/10.1038/519013a] [PMID: 25739606]

[65] Cdc.gov [homepage on internet]. United States. Severe outcomes among patients with Coronavirus disease 2019 (COVID-19) [updated on 27 Mar 2020]. Available from: https://www.cdc.gov/mmwr/volumes/69/wr/pdfs/mm6912e2-H.pdf

[66] Analysis on 54 Mortality Cases of Coronavirus Disease 2019 in the Republic of Korea from January 19 to March 10, 2020. J Korean Med Sci 2020; 35(12): e132. [http://dx.doi.org/10.3346/jkms.2020.35.e132] [PMID: 32233161]

[67] Niu S, Tian S, Lou J, *et al.* Clinical characteristics of older patients infected with COVID-19: A descriptive study. Arch Gerontol Geriatr 2020; 89: 104058. [http://dx.doi.org/10.1016/j.archger.2020.104058] [PMID: 32339960]

[68] Wang C, Pan R, Wan X, *et al.* Immediate Psychological Responses and Associated Factors during the Initial Stage of the 2019 Coronavirus Disease (COVID-19) Epidemic among the General Population in China. Int J Environ Res Public Health 2020; 17(5): 1729. [http://dx.doi.org/10.3390/ijerph17051729] [PMID: 32155789]

[69] Meng H, Xu Y, Dai J, Zhang Y, Liu B, Yang H. Analyze the psychological impact of COVID-19 among the elderly population in China and make corresponding suggestions. Psychiatry Res 2020; 289: 112983. [http://dx.doi.org/10.1016/j.psychres.2020.112983] [PMID: 32388175]

[70] Hsph.harvard.edu [homepage on internet], China: Harvard T.H. Chan School of Public Health [updated on July 2020], Coronavirus news. Available from: https://www.harvard.edu/coronavirus

[71] Weforum.org/agenda [homepage on internet], Covid-19 is hurting children's mental health. [updated on May 2020]. Available from: https://www.weforum.org/agenda/2020/05/covid-19-is-hurt-ng-childrens-mental-health/ 2020.

[72] 2020. Ewa.org [homepage on internet], Shock, rear, and fatalism: as coronavirus prompts colleges to close, students grapple with uncertainty. [updated on Mar 2020]. Available from: https://www.chronicle.com/article/shock-fear-and-fatalism-as-coronavirus-p-ompts-colleges-to-close-students-grapple-with-uncertainty/ 2020.

[73] Wagner KD. Addressing the experience of children and adolescents during the COVID-19 pandemic. J Clin Psychiatry 2020; 81: 20. [http://dx.doi.org/10.4088/JCP.20ed13394]

[74] Bussières EL, Malboeuf-Hurtubise C, Meilleur A, *et al.* Consequences of the COVID-19 Pandemic on Children's Mental Health: A Meta-Analysis. Front Psychiatry 2021; 12: 691659. [http://dx.doi.org/10.3389/fpsyt.2021.691659] [PMID: 34925080]

[75] Zhou SJ, Zhang LG, Wang LL, *et al.* Prevalence and socio-demographic correlates of psychological health problems in Chinese adolescents during the outbreak of COVID-19. Eur Child Adolesc Psychiatry 2020; 29(6): 749-58. [http://dx.doi.org/10.1007/s00787-020-01541-4] [PMID: 32363492]

[76] Son C, Hegde S, Smith A, Wang X, Sasangohar F. Effects of COVID-19 on College Students' Mental Health in the United States: Interview Survey Study. J Med Internet Res 2020; 22(9): e21279. [http://dx.doi.org/10.2196/21279] [PMID: 32805704]

[77] Unicef.org [homepage on internet], Impact of COVID-19 on poor mental health in children and young people 'tip of the iceberg'. [updated on Oct 2021]. Available from: https://www.unicef.org/press-releases/impact-covid-19-poor-mental-health-children-and-young-people-tip-iceberg

[78] Micelli E, Cito G, Cocci A, *et al.* Desire for parenthood at the time of COVID-19 pandemic: an insight into the Italian situation. J Psychosom Obstet Gynaecol 2020; 41(3): 183-90. [http://dx.doi.org/10.1080/0167482X.2020.1759545] [PMID: 32379999]

[79] Fairbrother N, Young AH, Zhang A, Janssen P, Antony MM. The prevalence and incidence of perinatal anxiety disorders among women experiencing a medically complicated pregnancy. Arch Women Ment Health 2017; 20(2): 311-9.
[http://dx.doi.org/10.1007/s00737-016-0704-7] [PMID: 28032213]

[80] Berthelot N, Lemieux R, Garon-Bissonnette J, Drouin-Maziade C, Martel É, Maziade M. Uptrend in distress and psychiatric symptomatology in pregnant women during the coronavirus disease 2019 pandemic. Acta Obstet Gynecol Scand 2020; 99(7): 848-55.
[http://dx.doi.org/10.1111/aogs.13925] [PMID: 32449178]

[81] Lebel C, MacKinnon A, Bagshawe M, Tomfohr-Madsen L, Giesbrecht G. Elevated depression and anxiety symptoms among pregnant individuals during the COVID-19 pandemic. J Affect Disord 2020; 277: 5-13.
[http://dx.doi.org/10.1016/j.jad.2020.07.126] [PMID: 32777604]

[82] Chen H, Guo J, Wang C, *et al.* Clinical characteristics and intrauterine vertical transmission potential of COVID-19 infection in nine pregnant women: a retrospective review of medical records. Lancet 2020; 395(10226): 809-15.
[http://dx.doi.org/10.1016/S0140-6736(20)30360-3] [PMID: 32151335]

[83] Un.org/en [homepage on internet]. United Nations. Make the prevention and redress of violence against women a key part of national response plans for COVID-19. 2020. Available from: https://www.un.org/en/un-coronavirus-communications-team/make-prevention-and-r-dress-violence-against-women-key-part

[84] Bradley NL, DiPasquale AM, Dillabough K, Schneider PS. Health care practitioners' responsibility to address intimate partner violence related to the COVID-19 pandemic. CMAJ 2020; 192(22): E609-10.
[http://dx.doi.org/10.1503/cmaj.200634] [PMID: 32357996]

[85] Npr.org. [homepage on internet]. Global lockdowns resulting in horrifying surge in domestic violence, U.N. warns. [updated on 6 Apr 2020]. Available from: https://www.npr.org/sections/coronavirus-liv--updates/2020/04/06/827908402/global-lockdowns-resulting-in-horrifying-surge-in--omestic-violence-u-n-warns

[86] Oecd.org [homepage on internet]. Addressing femicide in the context of rampant violence against women in latin America. Available from: https://www.oecd.org/gender/data/addressing-femicide--n-the-context-of-rampant-violence-against-women-in-latin-america.htm

[87] Druss BG. Addressing the COVID-19 pandemic in populations with serious mental illness. JAMA Psychiatry 2020; 77(9): 891-2.
[http://dx.doi.org/10.1001/jamapsychiatry.2020.0894] [PMID: 32242888]

[88] Dubey S, Biswas P, Ghosh R, *et al.* Psychosocial impact of COVID-19. Diabetes Metab Syndr 2020; 14(5): 779-88.
[http://dx.doi.org/10.1016/j.dsx.2020.05.035] [PMID: 32526627]

[89] Un.org [homepage on internet], United Nations. International Migration 2020 Highlights. [updated on 15 Jan 2021]. Available from: https://www.un.org/en/desa/international-migration-2020-highlights

[90] Unhcr.org [homepage on internet]. United Nations. UNHCR—Refugee Statistics. [Updated on 10 Nov 2021]. https://www.unhcr.org/refugee-statistics

[91] Satinsky E, Fuhr DC, Woodward A, Sondorp E, Roberts B. Mental health care utilisation and access among refugees and asylum seekers in Europe: A systematic review. Health Policy 2019; 123(9): 851-63.
[http://dx.doi.org/10.1016/j.healthpol.2019.02.007] [PMID: 30850148]

[92] Scott J. Homelessness and mental illness. Br J Psychiatry 1993; 162(3): 314-24.
[http://dx.doi.org/10.1192/bjp.162.3.314] [PMID: 8453425]

[93] Schreiter S, Bermpohl F, Krausz M, *et al.* The prevalence of mental illness in homeless people in Germany. Dtsch Arztebl Int 2017; 114(40): 665-72. [http://dx.doi.org/10.3238/arztebl.2017.0665] [PMID: 29070426]

CHAPTER 6

A Comprehensive Case Study Based On The Diversified Impacts Of COVID-19 On Children's Lives, Education And Overall Development

Faiza Ali[1,*], **Angila Shahab**[2] and **Jagrati Sharma**[1]

[1] *Department of Chemistry, Isabella Thoburn College, Lucknow-226007, Uttar Pradesh, India*

[2] *Department of Biosciences, Jamia Milia Islamia, New Delhi-110025, India*

Abstract: The impact of the COVID-19 pandemic on children is a developing worry. The United Nations and its agencies (the World Health Organization and UNICEF), the Indian Association for Child and Adolescent Mental Health, and India's National Institute of Mental Health and Neuroscience all warn of the pandemic's broader effects on children and call for immediate action to help children around the world. The pandemic had an impact on children's physical, mental, social, and psychological well-being in every way. The vulnerable group of children was severely deprived of nutrition and protection, and the pandemic's protracted stress-triggered mental health, which requires prompt intervention. Children who dropped out of school, particularly in rural regions, were at a higher risk of child marriage, child labour, and teen pregnancies. Based on the research, the current chapter highlights the influence of COVID-19 on the lives, education, and general development of children aged 4 to 17, in India. The authors were able to examine the pandemic's effects on children's lives using the snowball sampling approach in conjunction with peer-reviewed research, reports, and government publications published between January 2020 and November 2021. The findings revealed a negative trend in temperamental qualities such as sadness (82.5%) & nervosity (73.5%) that accelerated during the pandemic compared to pre-pandemic years. Also, children faced difficulties in receiving online education (53.6%). The chapter also highlighted the vulnerability of certain groups of children and presented numerous examples and recommendations that should be implemented as quickly as possible to mitigate the pandemic's negative impacts on children.

Keywords: Children, Child Labour, Child Marriage, COVID-19, e-Learners, e-Learning, Government, Impact, India, Mental Health, Neuroscience, Nutrition, Online Education, Pandemic, Psychological, Rural, Sadness, Snowball Sampling, Teen Pregnancies, Temperamental.

* **Corresponding author Faiza Ali**: Department of chemistry, Isabella Thoburn College, Lucknow-226007, Uttar Pradesh, India: E-mail: faizatahawwarali@gmail.com

Alfred J. Lawrence & Tahmeena Khan (Eds.)

INTRODUCTION

The World Health Organization (WHO) Director-General declared the outbreak of coronavirus disease (COVID-19) a Public Health Emergency of International Concern on 30 January 2020, followed by a loud and clear alarming declaration of COVID-19 as a global pandemic on 11 March 2020 [1]. The virus reported its early emergence from Wuhan, China, in late December 2019 [2]. The potential zoonotic formidable disease dispersed and expanded globally within a few months. In no time, the virus gripped its full potential and plunged economies into recession [3]. Stringent lockdowns and closure of all non-essential services were imposed throughout the globe. It becomes important to document the effects of the pandemic on the lives of the most vulnerable population, children. Forty-one per cent of India's population is under the age of 18, and the impact of a global pandemic on them cannot be underestimated [4]. The coronavirus illness (COVID-19) has a wide range of effects on children's physical, mental, social, and psychological health. These effects are not restricted not only to children's health and well-being; they also affect many aspects of their lives, including academics, protection, and security [5]. Many children have been deprived of physical contact with their friends, peers, and classmates as a result of the lockdown. Due to a lack of socialisation, they are more likely to lose their cool and become agitated and upset [5]. Children as young as five years old have had access to mobile phones for e-learning as a result of the shift in educational style [6]. The increased use of mobile phones and social networking sites increases the likelihood of becoming more absorbed in online amusement than academics [6]. Agencies have raised concerns that the pandemic's increased anxiety and stress on families may lead to an intensification of mental health problems in children [7]. COVID-19-positive children who are isolated, children of COVID-19-positive parents, and children who have lost one or both parents due to COVID-19 have a tough time coping with mental health concerns [8]. To feel a feeling of normalcy, such children must be helped by mental health service professionals, parents, and counsellors [8]. Furthermore, the pandemic's negative consequences are not distributed evenly. They are proven to be the most harmful to children in the poorest countries and neighbourhoods, as well as those who are already disadvantaged or vulnerable [9]. Also, no confirmed and tested vaccines are available to protect children from the fatal coronavirus [10]. the risk is amplified. Our comprehensive case study covers all the impacts faced by children due to this universal crisis. It is hard to fathom the exact prolonged effects but undoubtedly the pandemic has already affected the lives of children from almost all the spheres. With increased risks of exploitation, abuse and violence, deprivation from education, poverty driven lack of resources, upending physical and mental health, school closures, social isolation, uncertainty, fear and several other factors have bought up the lives of children to the shores of profound adverse experiences, consequences and impacts [11]. Long term broad ranging socio-economic and humanitarian impacts of the pandemic on children is highly likely to occur [11]. If not directly, indirectly the rippling effects of several deprivations will continue to harm children for a long time from today. Urgent actions and policies are needed to put forward for children at the forefront of preparedness, prevention and response to COVID-19 to ensure overall growth, development and well-being of children for all today and for the long term.

Data And Methodology

A study was undertaken using an online questionnaire-based survey titled "COVID-19 in context with children's lives, education, and overall development" to learn about the many implications of the COVID-19 pandemic on children's (aged 4-17) lives, academics, and overall well-being. The questionnaire was created with the help of prominent teachers and students from various age groups to cover all aspects of the influence. The study was carried out following the Helsinki Declaration's guidelines. A questionnaire survey is a simple and inexpensive approach to collecting information from a specific group. Furthermore, the data gathered by the questionnaire is simple to interpret and evaluate. The study location was Northern India, but the questionnaire was disseminated openly on several social media sites to allow for snowball sampling. A total of 412 responses were approved because they met the criteria for inclusion, which was based on the age of the children (4-17 years). The survey's questions were created to acquire a sense of how the activity pattern, behaviour, and temperamental features, as well as the impact on schooling, changed during the COVID-19 pandemic compared to the pre-pandemic pattern. Children of various schools across India belonging to class groups 1-12 (Fig. **1**) actively participated in the survey.

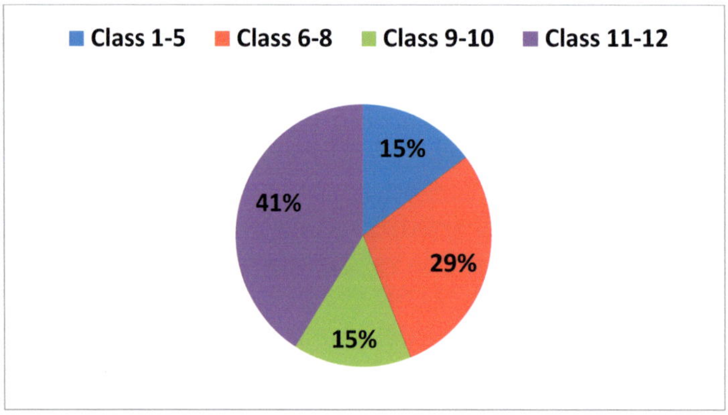

Fig. (1). % of children from various class groups who took part in the survey.

DIVERSIFIED IMPACT OF COVID-19 ON CHILDREN: POSITIVE AND NEGATIVE ASPECTS

A large number of studies and reports show how the pandemic can have long-term and far-reaching consequences on the present as well as the future of children [12]. It is anticipated that the impacts may worst hit the children who belong to already poor families, and disabled and displaced groups of children [12].

Among all this chaos, some positive impacts are also studied. The weightage may not be proportionate, but it would not be just to only state the heavy negative impacts. Our chapter has tried to cover the majority of impacts on different groups of children during the global crisis.

Positive Impacts

Physical

Quality Time with Family

The crisis can be viewed from an optimistic approach as it gave children some quality time at home with family. Since a home is known to be one of the best practical places to learn life skills, that, too, in a quite different situation of the pandemic, has enhanced the growth and development of children in several spheres [13].

Indulgence in More Indoor Activities

Observations show that during the lockdown period, families with proper education and awareness have completely tried to keep a consistent routine for children, especially by making them engage in maximum indoor activities. From contributing to daily chores of laundry, cooking, and cleaning, children had more time playing, fun reading, resting and playing board games. One main reason why children were made to pay attention to such activities was to deviate from video games and strategically decrease their screen time [14]. The majority (82.28%) (n=339) of children were involved in different kinds of physical activities during the pandemic for 1-2 hours on a daily basis (Fig. **2**).

Learning New Skills and Brain Booster Activities

The period of isolation has also helped children develop new skills which earlier due to heavy school and academic schedules they never thought to opt for or try. Space and free time somewhere helped children to find their hidden hobbies and interests [15]. Children who have access to online digital aids and other online distance learning programs are likely to get benefitted in the coming time. Children have become more friendly with technology-based learning.

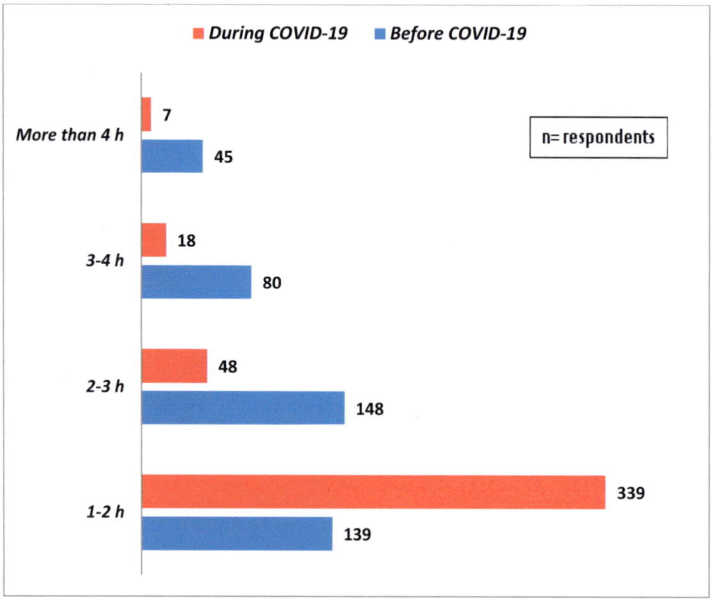

Fig. (2). Time (hours) spent on physical activity before and during the COVID-19 pandemic.

Psychological and Behavioural

Enhanced Ability to Face New Sudden Challenges

Our generation and its children were in no way familiar with the pandemic and its heavy consequences. Dealing with such a new problematic situation was not at all easy for anyone, but when it came to children, there was lots of uncertainty. Early school closures and break from all fixed routines somewhere was all fun and enjoyable for children. But with time, as the pandemic held its grip, tight waves of shock, fear, anxiety and trauma were spread all over. The point to discuss is that in such times a large proportion of children have shown enhanced abilities to deal and cope up and a new sense of responsibilities, active involvement, collaboration and accountability.

Enhanced Sense of Humanity and Empathy

Spending time with family and continuing to be in touch with some of the other people suffering, whether friends, relatives or colleagues, have developed a sense of humanity and empathy in many children. They have learned to handle emotions and started to value human life and health.

Social

New Opportunities Beyond Home and Schools

No one can deny that school closures and breaks from present-day hectic school schedules and private separate tuitions have provided children ample time to invest in their field of interest. With the help and support of parents, children have taken up active participation in art, music, dance and other such creative pursuits to maintain their mental health and well being [16].

Greater Awareness and Development

Complete constrained environment and unfamiliar circumstances enabled the young minds to develop more curiosity [17]. No matter what educational background children belonged to, they tried to learn more about all the biological information about viruses, the history of previous pandemics, and ways to survive. All at their level but an overall sense of awareness is seen in children.

Better Participation in Webinars and Other Social Online Interactions

The pandemic period flushed with lots of online programs, webinars, and even online social gatherings is seen to be a common thing during this time. Children are observed to have better participation in such initiatives. Sitting inside the home, children have completed several online courses, and volunteered to share their personal experiences of the pandemic times, their stories of patience and perseverance, which overall inspire and light up hope in many other juvenile hearts.

Value of Mother Nature and Planet Health

Early COVID-19 contagion when caused a nationwide lockdown in India from March 24th to 14th April, which later extended up to 3rd of May; studies show that in almost 88 cities, the pollution drastically reduced according to official data of CPCB [18]. To everyone's awe, such studies also forced little brains to think about their planet in consideration. Children learned more about the planet's health. They watched more nature, and wildlife and appreciated it [19].

Negative Impacts

Physical

Negative Changes in Daily Habits

Over the past several months' a tremendous decrease is observed in the physical health Of children. Multitudes of chronic diseases like diabetes, obesity, cardiovascular diseases are major consequences of physical inactivity due to constrained environments during a pandemic [20]. Overburdening of online classes, homework, and social media usage has overall caused a heavy increment in screen time of children making them more prone to weak eyesight. The long period of confinement pushed children towards addiction to internet usage and social media time passed, which resulted in more cases of abuse and vulnerability during the period. Considerable growth is observed in time spent on televisions or other OTT platforms (Fig. **3**) by children. 33.25% (n=137) of children were seen to exceed 3 hours. Reduced cardiorespiratory health [21], improper nutrition [22], and irregular sleep-wake cycles [23], have affected the overall health of children both physically and mentally.

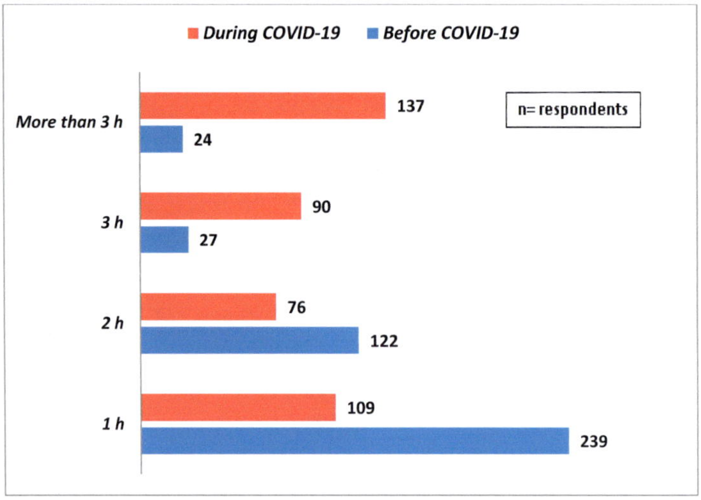

Fig. (3). Time (hours) spent watching T.V. /OTT before and during the COVID-19 pandemic.

Decreased Productivity

Lack of a healthy competitive environment, extremely limited outdoor exposure and constrained surroundings had an overall negative impact on the psychological well-being of children [24]. 57.76% of children reported an increase in distractions during the pandemic period (Fig. **4**). The lockdown started as fun for many children but further as the situation worsened, children were seen to be lazy and no more interested in many activities.

Lack of Personal Space

The adverse shift from physical learning at school to e-learning at home has forced children to face huge challenges. Several households with more family members suffered problematic situations due to limited personal space available in homes. Limited resources to attend online classes, disturbances due to family, and other household activities created a mess for children while attending classes. As a result, some children lost interest and were found to be missing their classes.

Deteriorated Health and Inadequate Nutrition

With the lost livelihood of parents or caregivers, closed markets, inadequate supply and price hikes, nutritious food was something very difficult for such families to afford. In several interrelated ways, covid has several concerning consequences for children. Not being able to access healthcare delivery, medicine and proper first aid, these factors disproportionately resulted in deteriorated health of children.

Physiological and Behavioural

Emotional Reactivity due to Stress

As compared to grown-ups, children and adolescents had a greater impact on social and behavioural development during the pandemic and lockdown. Increased cases of irritability, clinging behaviours and inattention are common in children [25]. 59.7% (n=246) children were seen to have quarrelsome attitudes and 53.15% (n=219) displayed self-centred traits during the pandemic (Fig. **4**).

Anxiety and Fear of Illness

Impacts seem to be more concerning when children face complete social isolation. No access to important facilities like counselling, guidance and support neither at school nor in families with much awareness has developed serious anxiety issues and an improper fear of illness. 73.5% of children were seen to be nervous, while 82.5% stated sadness in the survey (Fig. **4**). In a time when well-developed adults find it hard to maintain their mental health, the pandemic's far-reaching consequences on children are enough to haunt our imaginations.

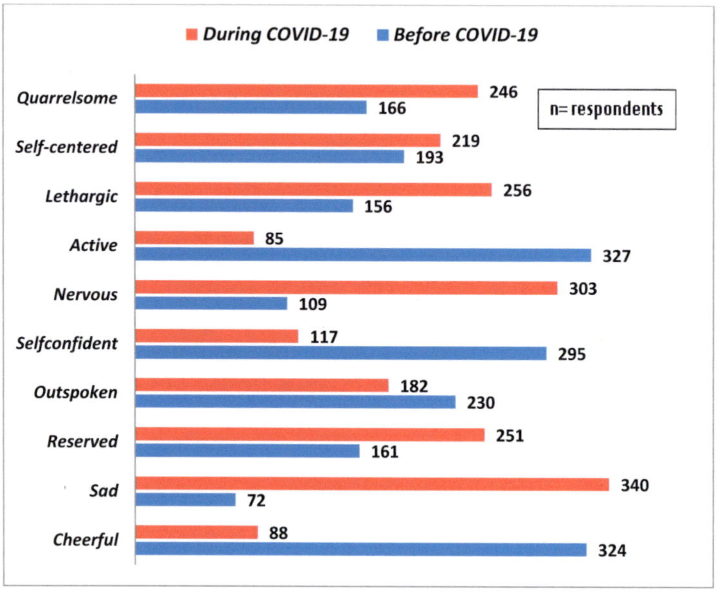

Fig. (4). Changes in temperamental traits in the child during COVID-19 pandemic as compared to pre-pandemic times.

Secondary Psychological Disorders

Due to sudden changes in the environment and enforced lockdown, children with special needs have encountered several difficulties. Lack of counselling, healthy interactions, unavailability of resources has negatively impacted the development of such children. 1 out of 6 children within the age group of 2-8 is seen to have special needs [26]. Autism, learning disability, OCD, cerebral palsy, ADHD are some to mention. 0.25%-0.4% of children and adolescents are estimated to be suffering from Obsessive-compulsive disorder. These children are suspected to be the worst-hit [26]. Living inside homes during lockdown complexes is the situation for children with Attention Deficit Hyperactivity Disorder (ADHD). To not touch things, following a list of rules and regulations to not get infected has resulted in hyperactivity, high pulse rates and therefore their health [27]. Children with autism easily get irritated and exasperated while facing new situations and conditions. Handling such children has also increased the challenge for parents due to the increased risk of self-harm [28].

Emotional Instability

Reduced well being and clear indications of stress are seen in children by unusual behaviours like unnecessary crying, breaking objects in anger, screaming and even bed wetting in some. 52.42% of respondents marked gradual growth in worry and anxiety issues while 55.58% of children were seen to be short-tempered during the pandemic span (Fig. **5**). An instinctual survival behaviour is observed due to panic buying in times of distress [29]. Among teenagers, a rise in hoarding behaviour is also observed [30]. The demise of loved ones, caregivers and deterioration in the health of family members or self have bought up children on the shores of hopelessness. Uncertainty, fear and nightmares are found to be common in the respective age group [31].

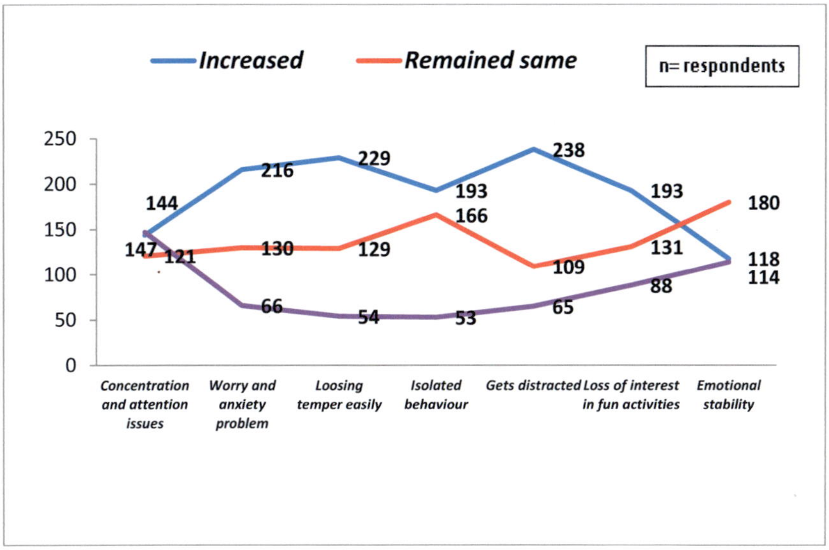

Fig. (5). Changes in the behaviour of children during the COVID-19 pandemic, compared to pre-pandemic times.

Social

Poverty

A large number of households, due to the pandemic and lockdown, lost their income and the majority of families reported heavy trouble paying even for their basic needs, including medical supplies, food, essential household services [32]. Poverty has accelerated negative parenting, child abuse, reduced psychosocial well being and heavy stress conditions.

From the hardship of crisis and severe loss of income, social protection could have acted as an insulation for the cause but due to its improper implementation as a side effect children are subjected to abuse, labour, kinds of harm and exploitation.

Child Abuse

Households dealing with economic shocks during the pandemic are more prone to cases of child abuse. The overall stressful environment, heavy household chores burden, caring duties and several other factors have severely affected the mental health and well being of children. Due to the partial functioning of legal and preventive organizations children were unable to express and report [33]. Since the lockdown began an increase in the calls received on the helpline for children was reported by 'CHILDLINE 1098' India's Deputy Director. This data specifies high rates of child abuse in their own homes [34]

Increased Risk of Child Exploitation

About 40 million children in India, among a total of approximate 472 million children population are severely impacted [35]. Children with disabilities, marginalized children, children living in conflict, deprived and displaced children seem to pay a higher consequence cost than other groups of children [36]. For girls in particular, school closures and no access to several items and services which earlier they used to get from school and organizations somewhere can act as catalysts to child marriages, abuse and labour (Fig. **6**).

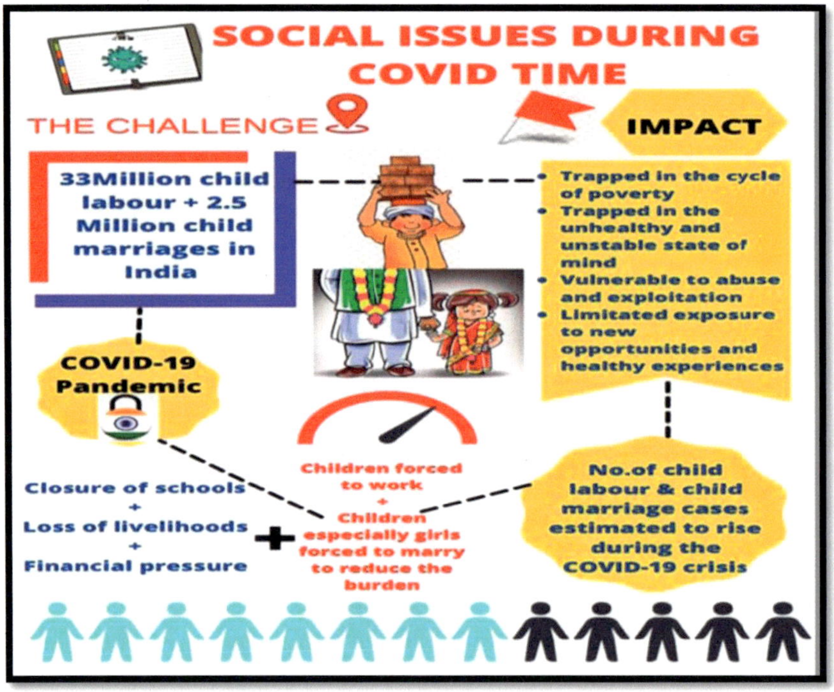

Fig. (6). Social issue enhancement during COVID-19 pandemic.

Effects on Education

The study reveals that two-thirds of parents and caregivers reported no contact from teachers after school closures with them or their children [37]. 8 out of 10 children felt they were learning nothing or just inadequate [37]. In rural areas, problems such as the increased burden of domestic chores partially more on girls than boys, increased duties on children towards their sibling, not being able to access learning materials, meals and other sanitary essentials which earlier were provided by schools, increased. All such factors paid heavy duty on children clashing with their right to education.

Increased School Dropouts

Children in bulk were seen to drop school and opt for paid work even when their little age doesn't allow them to. A great fall in adoption rate from offline to online classes is studied. Poor economic family conditions forced children from 6-18 age groups either to get enrolled in government schools having fewer fees (Table **1**) or to drop schools and search for paid work. Children who were infected with the virus were worst hit when they even lost their little income accompanying poor immunity and high medical expenses. The condition forced families to go into debt which not only shadows the child's present but also an uncertain future.

Table 1. Presents enrollment statistics from the ASER 2020 sample for several age groups. These figures show that more than 60% of all children in the 6-14 age range are enrolled in government schools, while nearly 30% are enrolled in private schools. [Source: Annual Status of Education Report (Rural) 2020, Wave 1, October 28, 2020] [38].

Age Group and Sex	Private	Government	Not in School	Others	Total
Age 6-14 All	28.8	65.8	4.6	0.8	100
Age 7-16 All	28.6	65.5	5.2	0.7	100
Age 7-10 All	30.5	64.3	4.4	0.8	100
Age 11-14 All	27.4	68.0	3.9	0.7	100
Age 15-16 All	27.3	62.1	9.9	0.6	100
Age 7-10 Girls	27.0	68.1	4.1	0.8	100
Age 11-14 Girls	23.5	71.9	3.9	0.7	100
Age 15-16 Girls	24.8	62.1	11.1	0.5	100
Age 7-10 Boys	33.6	60.9	4.7	0.8	100
Age 11-14 Boys	30.9	64.5	3.9	0.7	100
Age 15-16 Boys	29.7	60.8	8.8	0.8	100

COVID-19 PANDEMIC, E-LEARNING & CHILDREN

As the number of illnesses caused by COVID-19 infections grew at an alarming rate, the Indian government implemented a nationwide lockdown on 25th March 2020, suspending all essential &non-essential services, including educational institutions, to break the chain of infection [39]. As a result, it becomes vital to document its impact on students' lives and academic careers. Socioeconomic implications and mitigation measures that may unwittingly inflict more harm than good have an impact on all children, regardless of age or country of origin [40]. This outbreak is not predominantly impacting children. However, children are the risk of becoming its most significant victims, as the lives of children are dramatically impacted [41]. Education establishments have been obliged to adapt to e-learning to reduce the spread of the corona virus. Even though this quick shift poses obstacles, educational venues are readily available. The sudden closing of schools and colleges as a result of COVID-19 caused the government to push for the adoption of e-learning [42].

Virtual Learning: Promises and Challenges

With the help of virtual learning methods and educational materials in a classroom, numerous advantages like providing a class with more hands-on learning opportunities, using a variety of instructional techniques, improving student focus and understanding, and enhancing period for lecturers. The flexibility and ability to cross long distances are two main advantages of e-lea--ning. Schools and online platforms have prepared for a pandemic by rapidly digitizing their educational operations. Aside from their educational and economic functions, colleges play a variety of other tasks [43].

With the COVID-19 pandemic, it is becoming evident that the educational system is vulnerable to external threats. During this pandemic, students may suffer greatly in the following areas:

i. Racial, economic, and resource inequalities may have an impact on scholar academic performance; and
ii. The majority of teachers were unable to effectively give high-quality instruction remotely [44]. Some major problems faced by students (survey participants) while receiving online education are discussed in Table **2**.

Some of the challenges of virtual schools are; Students under-perform, technology is trying to exchange teachers, children miss out on social aspects, there's a low engagement of scholars, the high dropout rate of young girls and poor children, low completion, low retention rates and therefore the list goes on. The main challenge faced by students who cannot appear for their board examinations amid a pandemic.COVID-19 has also caused a shutdown of schools as well as economic suffering owing to loss of living, majorly in rural areas. High dropout rates and no enrollment in schools can be seen among young girls and poor children [45]. ASER 2020 investigated if this exceptional scenario has resulted in changes in rural India's academic enrolment trends (Table **3**).

Table 2. Table representing the problem faced by students in receiving an online education.

Problems faced by students in receiving online education. (Total responses= 333)		
Problems	**%**	**Respondents**
Lack of smartphones	9.9	33
Lack of stable internet connection	15.9	53
Poor understanding of topics	15.9	53
Poor concentration	13.8	46
Stress to eyes	26.1	87
Constant back and neck pain	4.5	15
Lack of self-confidence	1.5	5
Lack of competitive spirit among students	6.3	21
Less exposure to new opportunities	2.1	7

Table 3. Enrollment statistics from the ASER 2020 sample by age group and sex for Children not enrolled in school, in 2018 and 2020. [Source: Annual Status of Education Report (Rural) 2020, Wave 1, October 28, 2020] [38].

AGE GROUP	% Children					
	ASER 2018			ASER 2020		
	Girls	**Boys**	**All**	**Girls**	**Boys**	**All**
Age 15-16	12.6	11.4	12.0	11.1	8.8	9.9
Age 11-14	3.6	2.9	3.2	3.9	3.9	3.9
Age 6-10	1.8	1.8	1.8	5.2	5.3	5.3
All	4.2	3.7	4.0	5.7	5.3	5.5

The Absence of Standardized Assessment Presents Challenges for Students during the Cancellation of Board Exams because of COVID-19

For those who attend school, the Class 10 board exams are usually the first major milestone on the road to a career. The Class 12 board exams, which are even more important than the previous ones, are up next. Both of these have been cancelled this year by major school boards across the country. The ongoing coronavirus pandemic compelled the decision. The board exams are critical for students hoping to gain admission to some of India's most prestigious public universities. The cancellation of exams came as a huge relief to many students who were worried about taking exams at a time when India was gripped by a deadly second wave of the COVID-19 pandemic. However, for students, this relief quickly gave way to anxiety. It was upbeat at first, but soon questions about the future and what would happen arose. This will have a knock-on effect on college admissions. There will very certainly be a large number of unqualified candidates who receive inflated grades. As a result, the fairness of college admissions processes that use board exam scores as consideration will be called into question. The cancellation of board exams without considering the long-term consequences implies that the country's education system will be making things up as it goes for at least the next year, if not longer. There are benefits as well as drawbacks to obtaining certification without taking an exam [46].

E-Learning Practices: Positive and Negative Aspects

Positive Aspects of E-learning

Offers opportunities

❖India's online education market holds enormous promises and presents numerous career options for the country's rapidly ageing population. The spread of low-cost electronic learning is made possible by increased Internet penetration and widespread acceptance of online courses by major employers. Learning through the internet is a newer method of education.

Quick learning

❖E-Learning is a method of delivering lessons quickly. Some of the reasons why e-Learning reduces learning time are as follows:

❖Lessons begin quickly and are completed in a single lecture. It allows various trainee programs and internship programs to be conducted. Students do not need to travel to the training location to take part in these programs, it saves time.

Environment and financial friendly

❖When compared to traditional methods of learning, eLearning is less expensive. Furthermore, studying at home saves you money on travel fees. E-learning is also beneficial for the environment because it reduces paper production, which reduces pollution. Because virtual learning is a paperless way of learning, it contributes significantly to environmental protection.

Fig. (7). Positive aspects of e-learning [46].

Negative Aspects of E-learning

Requires motivation and time management

In typical classrooms, there are various elements that constantly push students toward their learning objectives. Live engagement with teachers, extracurricular activities, and rigid schedules all help students stay on track during their studies. A lack of self-motivation is one of the key reasons why students fail to complete online courses.

Inaccessible to those who lack resources

Despite fast technological improvement, computer literacy rates remain far from optimal. As long as such disparities remain in society, online education will be unable to reach all citizens. We must see online learning as a supplement to, rather than a replacement for, traditional education instead.

Lacks social interaction

Because you no longer see your teachers and students face-to-face, e-learning is one of the leading causes of social isolation. There is little to no interaction.

Fig. (8). Negative aspects of e-learning [47].

E-learning practices largely comprise online learning *via* numerous courses available on the internet. Emails live lectures, and videoconferencing can all be accomplished *via* the internet. This allows all parties to voice their views on a particular problem and then further discuss it. They also supply static sites, such as printed course materials, for all attendees' use. One of the major benefits (Fig. **7**) of utilizing the internet is that most online sites feature hyperlinks that will transport you to another page, allowing you to access a wealth of information [43 - 47]. You can learn from the comfort of your own home with the various online courses available. While on the opposite side of the picture, E-Learning methods now used in education tend to cause reflection, distance, and a lack of engagement in participants.

Consequently, many students who spend major time online may start to show signs of increased stress, anxiety, and the tendency to think negatively. As a result of their lack of human contact, many students who spend a lot of time online may begin to exhibit signs of social isolation (Fig. **8**). When people are socially isolated and unable to communicate, it can lead to several mental health issues such as increased stress, anxiety, and a tendency to think negatively [47]. The onset of online education made learning easy for some, while it also created distraction and hurdles for some. (Fig. **9**) represents a comparative analysis of online vs. offline education modes in different learning aspects.

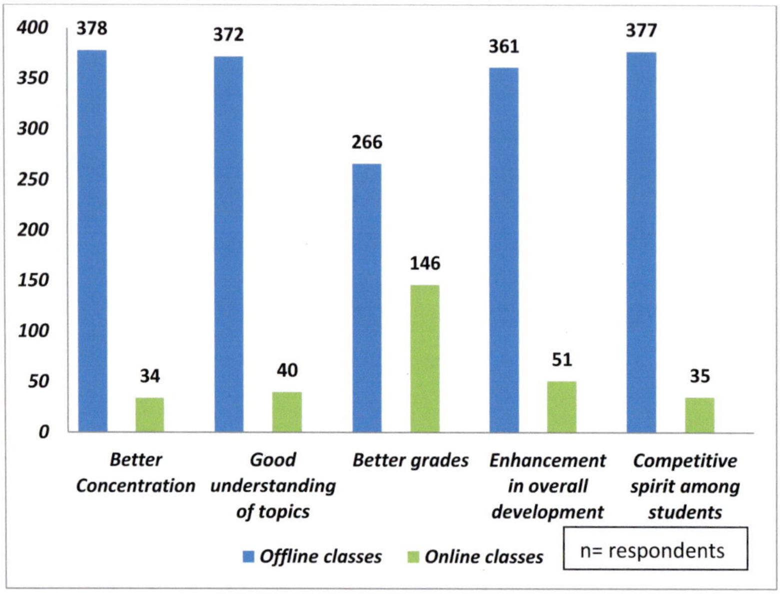

Fig. (9). A comparison of two modes of education, namely online and offline classes.

Impacts of E-Learning on Vulnerable (Rural & Poor children) Groups

Human rights are universal and applicable to everyone. The process of identifying vulnerable groups in the health and human rights sectors arose from the pressing reality on the ground, which resulted from the fact that there are there certain vulnerable and marginalized groups that do not have full access to a wide range of human rights, health and education. Many of these flaws render people more vulnerable to coronavirus infection, and many of the pandemic's impacts worsen the misery caused by the deprivations.

Access to the internet at home is heavily influenced by where you live and your socioeconomic status. Not having internet access now, during this pandemic, equates to not getting an education. People who live in slums, for example, are more likely to become infected and potentially very ill due to overcrowding and a lack of access to water and sanitation. Anyone whose income falls below the poverty threshold is considered poor and included among those who don't have access to resources.

It's also simple to help poor families cope with income losses during a pandemic, governments should increase existing cash transfer programmes (or add new ones if so required). However, we suggest that, in addition to a lack of sufficient income, other forms of deprivation demand equal attention. Domestic abuse, as well as discrimination in the health care system based on skin colour, sexual orientation, or migrant status, are deprivations that are aggravated during the pandemic. Cash transfers alone will not be enough to tackle these problematic practices. Cash transfers will not provide the type of training that children require to be successful at homeschooling. To construct an effective policy response, it is necessary to first identify the vulnerable populations and their needs. Children who live on the streets face significant vulnerabilities in normal times, as well as additional ones at this time. Some children may find themselves completely alone as a result of the death or illness of a sole caregiver. Many children's living conditions deteriorate as a result of their parents' financial difficulties. In the current climate, many people are having difficulty receiving care and School closures endanger the education of poor children [48].

Implications of COVID-19 on Education

The COVID-19 pandemic has caused unprecedented disruption across all industries, including education. In such a difficult time, society and industries have sought to counteract the pandemic's disruptions through "great decentralization," *i.e.*, work-from-home or work-from-anywhere. Similarly, online education is becoming more common in most colleges and universities. However, due to the digital divide in India, online education has some limitations. In this context, the government and other stakeholders should view the disruption caused by the pandemic as an opportunity to improve and modernize the public education system.

Although enrollment had increased during the previous two decades, millions of youngsters were already absent when the pandemic began. And when the schools reopen, many of them will be empty. Children from low-income homes, as well as teenage girls who are at high risk of pregnancy, are more vulnerable. The government system will be strained if more people choose public schools instead of private ones, especially in urban regions where new public-school construction has not kept pace with population growth. Some students will be unable to attend school because of transportation and financial issues. There is little chance that the demand for education from parents will decrease, which means that low-cost private schools will maintain their current market share for the foreseeable future but will have disastrous consequences for children as well as the millions of female teachers who work with them [49].

When possible, education should be continued through online courses. Companies should start offering customized packages as part of their services to enable free or subsidized Wi-Fi for educational purposes. If internet-based teaching isn't a possibility, more “traditional” methods, such as television or even radio, should be considered. Retired teachers and other persons could donate their time to provide coaching and mentoring to impoverished children and teens as part of the above-mentioned social protection [50].

VULNERABLE GROUPS OF CHILDREN AFFECTED BY COVID-19

Other vulnerable populations (Fig. **10**), in addition to poor children, suffered equally or even more during the COVID-19 pandemic. There is an immediate need for protection for them, as the long-term consequences could permanently harm their physical, mental and social well-being [51]. The different vulnerable groups include:

1. ***Poor Children & Slum Dwellers:*** A billion people live in slums or substandard dwellings with no access to appropriate sanitation [52]. They rely on communal sanitation procedures since they do not have access to piped water or sufficient hand-washing facilities at home. As a result, the risk of covid infection increases.
2. ***Child Refugees:*** Internally displaced children and children living in camps or crowded communities face similar issues. They are more likely to be denied social assistance and medical care, as well as have difficulty finding a safe place to live [53].
3. ***Children Who Lost their Parents due to the Pandemic:*** Children who have lost one or both of their parents during the COVID-19 pandemic felt a loss of protection and warrants special attention. According to the National Commission for the Protection of Child Rights, 3,621 children lost both parents to the pandemic between April 1, 2020, and June 5, 2021, 26,176 children lost one parent, and 274 children were abandoned [54].
4. ***Differently-Abled Children:*** The COVID-19 outbreak poses a threat to the well-being of children with disabilities on multiple levels, including education, health, social protection. It has caused enormous stress and disturbance in the lives of children who thrive on order and routine in normal conditions. Children with disabilities may require additional assistance in adjusting to these numerous changes and learning how to be safe. Many differently-abled children receive therapy care to help them improve their communication and social-emotional skills, as well as manage better at school and home [55]. These youngsters would now require further assistance in developing and maintaining new routines, as well as calming and coping abilities.

5. ***Children Living in Institutions/NGOs:*** Numerous non-governmental organizations work in the field of education and child development. They bring out-of-school youngsters to the classroom; reintroduce street children and young labourers to the educational system. This crisis made those children deprived of education and their basic needs who were part of these non-governmental organizations. Thousands of charitable organizations in India mobilized almost immediately to provide food, healthcare, information, monetary transfers, and transportation to those affected. However, these NGOs have been grappling with the pandemic's impact on their capacities and long-term viability. Many non-governmental organizations (NGOs) are in dire financial straits since the majority of cash and donations are being channelled to the COVID-19 pandemic and relief operations [56, 57].

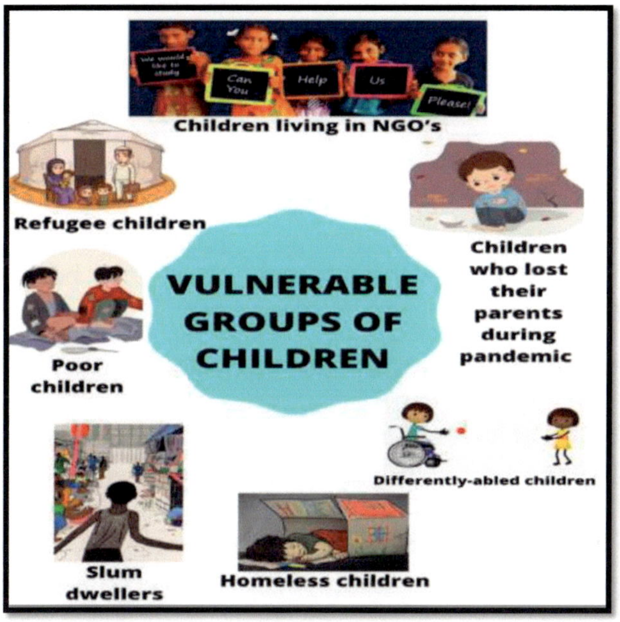

Fig. (10). Vulnerable group of children affected during the COVID-19 pandemic.

RECOMMENDATIONS AND EXEMPLARS

The COVID-19 pandemic is a curse for the entire planet, as it has caused a series of losses since its onset. The outbreak had a serious influence on children's mental, physical, and social well-being, and many students' academic careers were also damaged as a result. Due to the terrible scenario created by the COVID-19 pandemic, children from poor households suffered from hunger and severe financial hardship. There has to be a method to counteract it [57]. To tackle the horrible situation produced by the pandemic, new methods should be developed and implemented in addition to preventive measures. Because children are the most susceptible population, special and effective techniques must be developed and implemented to reduce the detrimental impact on them.

Following are some Recommendations and Policies that can be Devised to Help Children Afflicted by the COVID-19 Pandemic [58]

Reinforcing Food Assistance Programs

Food assistance programs are proposed by the national government in conjunction with non-governmental organizations (NGOs) and members of civil society to improve the nutritional well-being of citizens who would otherwise lack access to appropriate food for a healthy life. People suffered from financial and mental breakdowns, but poor families, who were the most vulnerable, also faced food shortages. As they began to suffer from malnutrition, the children in those homes became the primary perpetrators. To combat this situation, the government should strengthen various food assistance programs for affected children, such as the Integrated Child Development Service Program (ICDS), Special Nutrition Program (SNP), and Balwadi Nutrition Program, and a suitable body should be appointed to ensure proper food distribution to these children [59]. In addition, the mid-day food program in government schools should be reinstated to help afflicted children.

Initiatives To Alleviate Child Poverty And Relieve Financial Challenges

Children are regarded to be the most vulnerable category, yet children from low-income homes are more fragile. It is necessary to make attempts to safeguard and uplift them. State education departments should try to reduce their financial responsibilities by utilising loans and equated monthly installments (EMI) for school fees [60].

Increment Of Student-Teacher Interaction

The student-teacher interaction is declining with each passing day as a result of the shift from offline to online education. As a result, students are less engaged in attending lessons, and their academic performance suffers. Efforts should be made to address these issues. Teachers should be monitored, encouraged, and supported to contact students *via* phone calls, text messages, or safe home visits by the district and block education officers [61]. In regions where device access or internet connection is limited, the concept of open-air classrooms can be promoted.

Drive Re-enrollment Programs To Prevent Students From Dropping Out

Children in bulk were seen to drop school and opt for paid work even when their little age doesn't allow them to. Poor economic family conditions developed due to the pandemic and stringent lockdowns forced children from 6-18 age groups to drop schools and search for paid work. To counter-attack the situation, the state can hold virtual meetings with students and parents *via* phone calls or text messages, as well as in-person meetings, to prevent them from dropping out and to ensure their enrolment for the future academic year [62].

Assisting Students In Overcoming Large Learning Losses

The pandemic caused a significant shift in the learning spectrum, as well as changes in school systems, compared to pre-pandemic days. The abrupt transition from offline to online classes proved to be a hardship for the students. Some youngsters were unable to defend themselves against this challenge, and as a result, their academic performance suffered. To combat learning loss, states can work with ed-tech platforms or non-governmental organizations to establish a well-developed evaluation system that can track each child's progress. These assessment systems will assist government schools in determining a child's readiness [63].

Mitigating Mental Health Problems

The COVID-19 epidemic imposed a slew of issues that have ramifications for everyone, but especially for children and adolescents' mental health. Over 330 million children were stranded at home for two years. The prolonged isolation rendered them extremely susceptible, and the chances of their getting anxiety and depression, as well as suicidal tendencies, rose. Children should be encouraged to discuss their feelings with their family and friends to combat this difficulty. Early intervention can aid in the prevention of long-term repercussions [64]. Children should be engaged in creative activities such as playing and sketching when they are young. To feel cheerful and relaxed, children aged 10 to 17 can participate in some online beneficial classes or read some valuable novels.

Initiatives To Provide Smartphones To Less Privileged Students

Owing to the closure of schools due to the COVID-19 epidemic, education has shifted from offline to online. This move caused challenges for both students and teachers, but the less fortunate students, particularly those in rural areas who are financially and economically disadvantaged, could not afford smartphones or laptops to attend online classes [65]. As a result, they were forced to stop their study right then and there. If necessary steps are not taken to offer such learners facilities so that they can continue their education in either form, they will be left behind at every chance. Every state government can aid such children by providing smartphones or laptops. In such places, a stable internet connection should be installed so that students and teachers have no difficulties conducting and receiving online education [66].

CONCLUDING REMARKS

This extensive case study in India, based on information from research papers, government publications, and other reports, demonstrated how the COVID-19 pandemic had harmed the most vulnerable children. The global crisis influenced them not just because of the virus, but also because it affected them in many aspects of their lives, whether directly or indirectly [67]. The detrimental trend can be seen in temperamental traits as many children started to develop feelings of sadness (82.5%), nervousness (73.5%), distractions (58%), loss of interest in fun activities (47%) as compared to the pre-pandemic times. During the pandemic, many children were unable to meet the challenge of switching from offline to online education. Due to a lack of sufficient planning & resources, a slew of issues arose in front of the learners, such as lack of smartphones or laptops (33.3%), lack of stable internet connection (15.9%), stress to eyes (26.1%), lack of exposure to new opportunities (13.8%). The condition of learners in rural areas has gotten worse, as many of them have had to drop out of school due to financial difficulties and a lack of access to digital resources. As a result, many young children were obliged to work for pay to help their families improve their financial situation, resulting in the escalation of different social issues like child labour, child abuse and teenage pregnancies during the pandemic [67]. To defend this challenge, collective efforts of central and state governments in collaboration with several non-government organizations and private sectors are needed to mitigate the severe impact of the COVID-19 pandemic on children's well-being [68]. Social issues like child labour, child marriage, child abuse can be addressed under national adolescent health programmes [69, 70] and strict actions must be taken to irradiate such social issues.

CONSENT FOR PUBLICATION

Not applicable.

CONFLICT OF INTEREST

The authors declare no conflict of interest, financial or otherwise.

ACKNOWLEDGEMENTS

Declared none.

REFERENCES

[1] Cucinotta D, Vanelli M. WHO Declares COVID-19 a Pandemic. Acta Biomed 2020; 91(1): 157-60. [PMID: 32191675]

[2] Liu W, Zhang Q, Chen J, *et al.* Detection of COVID-19 in Children in Early January 2020 in Wuhan, China. N Engl J Med 2020; 382(14): 1370-1. [http://dx.doi.org/10.1056/NEJMc2003717] [PMID: 32163697]

[3] Thompson R. Pandemic potential of 2019-nCoV. Lancet Infect Dis 2020; 20(3): 280. [http://dx.doi.org/10.1016/S1473-3099(20)30068-2] [PMID: 32043978]

[4] https://unsdg.un.org/resources/policy-brief-impact-COVID-19-children

[5] https://data.unicef.org/COVID-19-and-children/

[6] Al-Mandhari A, Samhouri D, Abubakar A, Brennan R. Coronavirus Disease 2019 outbreak: preparedness and readiness of countries in the Eastern Mediterranean Region. East Mediterr Health J 2020; 26(2): 136-7. [http://dx.doi.org/10.26719/2020.26.2.136] [PMID: 32141588]

[7] Sheahan TP, Frieman MB. The continued epidemic threat of SARS-CoV-2 and implications for the future of global public health. Curr Opin Virol 2020; 40: 37-40. [http://dx.doi.org/10.1016/j.coviro.2020.05.010] [PMID: 32569751]

[8] https://unsdg.un.org/[homepage on the Internet]https://unsdg.un.org/resources/policy-brief-impa-t-COVID-19-children

[9] Kupferschmidt K, Cohen J. Will novel virus go pandemic or be contained? Science 2020; 367(6478): 610-1. [http://dx.doi.org/10.1126/science.367.6478.610] [PMID: 32029604]

[10] Swami nathan S . Episode #42 - Vaccines and children [Video]. World Health Organization 11 June 2021 | Science conversation . 2021.

[11] Tisdell CA. Economic, social and political issues raised by the COVID-19 pandemic. Econ Anal Policy 2020; 68: 17-28. [http://dx.doi.org/10.1016/j.eap.2020.08.002] [PMID: 32843816]

[12] Fenichel EP. Economic considerations for social distancing and behavioral based policies during an epidemic. J Health Econ 2013; 32(2): 440-51. [http://dx.doi.org/10.1016/j.jhealeco.2013.01.002] [PMID: 23419635]

[13] Denham SA. Relationships between Family Rituals, Family Routines, and Health. J Fam Nurs 2003; 9(3): 305-30. [http://dx.doi.org/10.1177/1074840703255447]

[14] Brooks SK, Webster RK, Smith LE, *et al.* The psychological impact of quarantine and how to reduce it: rapid review of the evidence. Lancet 2020; 395(10227): 912-20. [http://dx.doi.org/10.1016/S0140-6736(20)30460-8] [PMID: 32112714]

[15] Wang G, Zhang Y, Zhao J, Zhang J, Jiang F. Mitigate the effects of home confinement on children during the COVID-19 outbreak. Lancet 2020; 395(10228): 945-7. [http://dx.doi.org/10.1016/S0140-6736(20)30547-X] [PMID: 32145186]

[16] Brown GTL. Schooling Beyond COVID-19: An Unevenly Distributed Future. Frontiers in Education 2020; 5: 82. [http://dx.doi.org/10.3389/feduc.2020.00082]

[17] Cole M. What's Culture Got to Do With It? Educ Res 2010; 39(6): 461-70. [http://dx.doi.org/10.3102/0013189X10380247]

[18] https://www.pnas.org/content/118/17/e2022376118

[19] Sharma A, Balyan P. Air pollution and COVID-19: Is the connect worth its weight? Indian J Public Health 2020; 64(6) (Suppl.): 132. [http://dx.doi.org/10.4103/ijph.IJPH_466_20] [PMID: 32496243]

[20] Paffenbarger RS Jr, Hyde R, Wing AL, Hsieh C. Physical activity, all-cause mortality, and longevity of college alumni. N Engl J Med 1986; 314(10): 605-13. [http://dx.doi.org/10.1056/NEJM198603063141003] [PMID: 3945246]

[21] Dayton JD, Ford K, Carroll SJ, Flynn PA, Kourtidou S, Holzer RJ. The deconditioning effect of the COVID-19 pandemic on unaffected healthy children. Pediatr Cardiol 2021; 42(3): 554-9. [http://dx.doi.org/10.1007/s00246-020-02513-w] [PMID: 33394120]

[22] Ammar A, Brach M, Trabelsi K, *et al.* Effects of COVID-19 home confinement on eating behaviour and physical activity: results of the ECLB-COVID19 international online survey. Nutrients 2020; 12(6): 1583. [http://dx.doi.org/10.3390/nu12061583] [PMID: 32481594]

[23] Dellagiulia A, Lionetti F, Fasolo M, Verderame C, Sperati A, Alessandri G. Early impact of COVID-19 lockdown on children's sleep: a 4-week longitudinal study. J Clin Sleep Med 2020; 16(9): 1639-40. [http://dx.doi.org/10.5664/jcsm.8648] [PMID: 32620188]

[24] Lee J. Mental health effects of school closures during COVID-19. Lancet Child Adolesc Health, 2020; S2352-4642(20): 30109-7.

[25] Viner RM, Russell SJ, Croker H, *et al.* School closure and management practices during coronavirus outbreaks including COVID-19: a rapid systematic review. Lancet Child Adolesc Health 2020; 4(5): 397-404. [http://dx.doi.org/10.1016/S2352-4642(20)30095-X] [PMID: 32272089]

[26] https://www.cdc.gov/childrensmentalhealth/data.html

[27] Cortese S, Asherson P, Sonuga-Barke E, *et al.* ADHD management during the COVID-19 pandemic: guidance from the European ADHD Guidelines Group. Lancet Child Adolesc Health 2020; 4(6): 412-4. [http://dx.doi.org/10.1016/S2352-4642(20)30110-3]

[28] Children with autism and COVID-19. https://www.unicef.org/serbia/en/children-autism-and-CO-ID-19

[29] Arafat SY, Kar SK, Marthoenis M, Sharma P, Apu EH, Kabir R. Psychological underpinning of panic buying during pandemic (COVID-19). Psychiatry Res 2020 Jul; 289: 113061.

[30] Oosterhoff B, Palmer CA, Wilson J, Shook N. Adolescents' motivations to engage in social distancing during the covid-19 pandemic: associations with mental and social health. J Adolesc Health 2020 Aug; 67(2): 179-85.

[31] Jiao WY, Wang LN, Liu J, *et al.* Behavioral and emotional disorders in children during the COVID-19 epidemic. J Pediatr. PubMed 2020; 221: pp. 264-266.e1.

[32] https://resourcecente.savethechildren.net

[33] Singh S, Roy D, Sinha K, Parveen S, Sharma G, Joshi G. Impact of COVID-19 and lockdown On mental health of children and adolescents: A narrative review with recommendations. Psychiatry Res 2020; 293: 113429.

[34] https://economictimes.indiatimes.com/news/politics-and-nation/govt-helpline-receives-92000-calls-on-abuse-and-violence-in-11-days/articleshow/75044722.cms?utm_source=contentofinterest&utm_medium=text&utm_campaign=cppst

[35] Dalton L, Rapa E, Stein A. Protecting the psychological health of children through effective communication about COVID-19. Lancet Child Adolesc Health 2020; 4(5): 346-7. [http://dx.doi.org/10.1016/S2352-4642(20)30097-3] [PMID: 32243784]

[36] Rosenthal DM, Ucci M, Heys M, Hayward A, Lakhanpaul M. Impacts of COVID-19 on vulnerable children in temporary accommodation in the UK. Lancet Public Health 2020; 5(5): e241-2. [http://dx.doi.org/10.1016/S2468-2667(20)30080-3] [PMID: 32243776]

[37] Birla N. Mental health may hurt India to tune of $1.03 trillion; here's a dose for cos. Econ. TImes, India Times. 2019. [Cited: 30th October 2021]. Available from: https://economictimes.indiatimes.scom/magazines/panache/mental-health-may-hurt-india-to-tune-of-1-03-trillion-heres-a-dose-for-cos/articleshow/71045027.cms

[38] Annual Status of Education Report (Rural) 2020, Wave 1, October 28, 2020 [Cited: 31st October 2021]. Available from: http://img.asercentre.org/docs/ASER%202020/ASER%202020%20REPORT/aser2020fullreport.pdf

[39] Alan S, Greg S, Barbara F. Insights into accounting education in a COVID-19 world. Accn. Edu 2020; 5: 431-562.

[40] https://www.drishtiias.com/daily-updates/daily-news-editorials/education-in-post-covid-era

[41] https://unesdoc.unesco.org/ark:/48223/pf0000374702

[42] Abdelsalam M. Maatuk, Ebitisam K Elberkawi, Shadi Aljawarneh, Hasan Rashaideh, Hadeel Alharbi The COVID-19 pandemic and E-learning: challenges and opportunities from the perspective of students and instructors. Comput. High. Edu 2021; pp. 2-18.

[43] https://elearningindustry.com/advantages-and-disadvantages-of-elearning

[44] Soykan Emrah COVID-19 pandemic and online learning: the challenges and opportunities. Int. Lear. Envir 2020; pp. 4-6.

[45] https://talentedge.com/blog/scope-opportunities-online-learning-india

[46] https://achievevirtual.org/blog/parent-resources/parent-engagement-with-student-online-lear-ing-is-important

[47] https://e-student.org/disadvantages-of-e-learning/

[48] Covid-19 and social protection of poor and vulnerable groups in Latin America: a conceptual framework. IOP Publishing UNDP Latin America and the Caribbean 2020.

[49] IOP Publishing centre for global development https://www.cgdev.org/blog/six-ways-COVID-19--ill-shape-future-education.

[50] https://jamanetwork.com/journals/jamapediatrics/fullarticle/2766114

[51] https://data.unicef.org/COVID-19-and-children/

[52] https://www.unicef.org/coronavirus/agenda-for-action

[53] https://ec.europa.eu/research-and-innovation/en/horizon-magazine/how-vulnerable-groups-we-e-left-behind-pandemic-response

[54] https://www.socialscienceinaction.org/resources/COVID-19-impacts-of-the-pandemic-on-vul-erable-communities-in-india/

[55] https://www.thehindu.com/news/national/645-children-lost-their-parents-to-covid-from--pr-may-28-during-second-wave-wcd/article35468032.ece

[56] https://www.my.undp.org/content/malaysia/en/home/blog/2020/COVID-19-and-the-most-vulnerable-among-us.html?utm_source=EN&utm_medium=GSR&utm_content=US_UNDP_PaidSearch_Brand_English&utm_campaign=CENTRAL&c_src=CENTRAL&c_src2=GSR&gclid=Cj0KCQiA-eeMBhCpARIsAAZfxZA8ps7EJ9WL-BmNYJ8TyIwItTgcuNYqJUVaCAGpbW-M_9zWtNtEBJ

kaAm_DEALw_wcB

[57] https://www.oecd.org/coronavirus/policy-responses/combatting-COVID-19-s-effect-on-c-ildren-2e1f3b2f/

[58] https://data.unicef.org/COVID-19-and-children/

[59] https://www.unicef.org/coronavirus/agenda-for-action

[60] https://ec.europa.eu/research-and-innovation/en/horizon-magazine/how-vulnerable-groups-we-e-left-behind-pandemic-response

[61] https://www.socialscienceinaction.org/resources/COVID-19-impacts-of-the-pandemic-on-vul-erable-communities-in-india/

[62] https://www.thehindu.com/news/national/645-children-lost-their-parents-to-covid-from-apr-may-28-during-second-wave-wcd/article35468032.ece

[63] COVID-19 and the Most Vulnerable Among Us. https://www.my.undp.org/content/malaysia/en/home/blog/2020/COVID-19-and-the-most-vulnerable-among-us.html?utm_source=EN&utm_medium=GSR&utm_content=US_UNDP_PaidSearch_Brand_English&utm_campaign=CENTRAL&c_src=CENTRAL&c_src2=GSR&gclid=Cj0KCQiA-eeMBhCpARIsAAZfxZA8ps7EJ9WL-BmNYJ8TyIwItTgcuNYqJUVaCAGpbW-M_9zWtNtEBJkaAm_DEALw_wcB

[64] https://www.oecd.org/coronavirus/policy-responses/combatting-COVID-19-s-effect-on-c-ildren-2e1f3b2f/

[65] https://www.nasponline.org/resources-and-publications/resources-and-podcasts/school-safe-y-and-crisis/health-crisis-resources/helping-children-cope-with-changes-resulting-from-COVID-19

[66] Phillips DE, Bhutta ZA, Binagwaho A, *et al.* Learning from Exemplars in Global Health: a road map for mitigating indirect effects of COVID-19 on maternal and child health. BMJ Glob Health 2020; 5(7): e003430.
[http://dx.doi.org/10.1136/bmjgh-2020-003430] [PMID: 32737028]

[67] Perry HB, Dhillon RS, Liu A, *et al.* Community health worker programmes after the 2013–2016 Ebola outbreak. Bull World Health Organ 2016; 94(7): 551-3.
[http://dx.doi.org/10.2471/BLT.15.164020] [PMID: 27429495]

[68] Hadi A. Promoting health knowledge through micro-credit programmes: experience of BRAC in Bangladesh. Health Promot Int 2001; 16(3): 219-27.
[http://dx.doi.org/10.1093/heapro/16.3.219] [PMID: 11509457]

[69] Fore HH. A wake-up call: COVID-19 and its impact on children's health and wellbeing. Lancet Glob Health 2020; 8(7): e861-2.
[http://dx.doi.org/10.1016/S2214-109X(20)30238-2] [PMID: 32405458]

[70] Douglas M, Katikireddi SV, Taulbut M, McKee M, McCartney G. Mitigating the wider health effects of COVID-19 pandemic response. BMJ 2020; 369: m1557.
[http://dx.doi.org/10.1136/bmj.m1557]

CHAPTER 7

COVID-19 Vaccines: A Brief Review

Saman Raza[1,*]

[1] *Department of Chemistry, Isabella Thoburn College, Lucknow-226007, Uttar Pradesh, India*

Abstract: The advent of the COVID-19 pandemic in December 2019 was a defining moment in medical history that pushed the world into a state of uncertainty and fear. The virus was a new one, its effects on the human body were severe and its ever-growing spread across the globe soon became a major concern for everyone, drawing an extraordinary response from the scientific community, doctors, health workers and governments. The research was conducted on the structure and physiology of the virus as well as the human immune response to the virus, along with the development of testing, therapeutics, and vaccines occurring on an unprecedentedly short timescale. With support from governments and pharmaceutical companies, within a year of the worldwide outbreak of the disease, numerous vaccine candidates had emerged, and to date, eight World Health Organization-approved vaccines are being used on an emergency basis. In this concise review, the different types of vaccines have been described, along with the characteristics of the leading vaccines and a detailed discussion of the vaccines being used in India.

Keywords: Adenovirus, Adjuvant, Antibodies, Antigen, Approval, Attenuated, Covaxin, COVID-19, Covishield, Efficacy, Immune-response, Inactivated, mRNA, Pandemic, Pharmaceutical, Spike-protein, Sputnik-V, Vaccine, Viral-vector, Virus.

INTRODUCTION

While vaccines for several diseases, such as smallpox, measles, tetanus, influenza and polio, have been used worldwide for years, it is in times like the present, when the entire world is facing a novel pandemic for which no medicine is known yet, the significance of vaccines has increased manifold. Before discussing the different vaccines available for COVID-19, let us first understand what vaccines are and how they protect against diseases.

A vaccine can be defined as a suspension of weakened, killed, or fragmented microorganisms or toxins that is administered primarily to prevent disease [1].

* **Corresponding author Saman Raza**: Department of Chemistry, Isabella Thoburn College, Lucknow-226007, Uttar Pradesh, India: E-mail: samanmahek@gmail.com

Alfred J. Lawrence & Tahmeena Khan (Eds.)

A vaccine helps our immune system to recognize a pathogen (bacteria, virus, *etc.*) and prepare an immune response in the form of antibodies so that if the pathogen attacks the body later, it would be able to quickly respond and fight and destroy the disease-causing pathogen. This acquired immunity protects the vaccinated person from the severity of the disease and reduces fatality.

Vaccines are of several types based on the method of their formulation and mode of action [2]. The major types of vaccines are briefly discussed below (Fig. **1**).

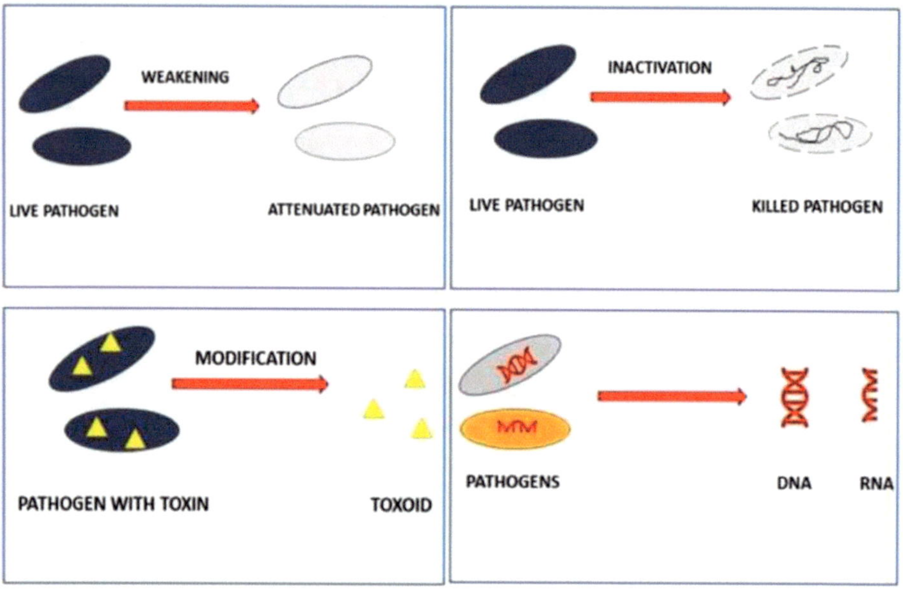

Fig. (1). Types of vaccines.

Live, Attenuated Vaccines

These use a weakened form of the disease-causing germs that have lost the ability to replicate in the body. This can be done by passing the virus through a series of non-human cell cultures, where it slowly loses its ability to replicate in human cells. When such a vaccine is taken, it cannot cause an infection as the virus cannot multiply, but being so similar to the actual pathogen, it can still cause an immune response. These vaccines are quite effective and provide longer-lasting immunity as they resemble the actual disease-causing pathogen the most. One concern regarding live vaccines is that they may undergo mutations and form a more virulent form of the pathogen [3]; although such an event is quite unlikely, it is kept in mind during vaccine preparation, and suitable steps are taken to avoid it. The disadvantage of such vaccines is that they cannot be given to people with a weakened immune system as they contain the weakened but live pathogen. Also, they have to be kept refrigerated and become difficult to use where such facilities are lacking [4].

Examples: Measles, mumps, rubella (MMR combined vaccine), chickenpox, influenza, and rotavirus vaccines.

Killed or Inactivated Vaccines

In these vaccines, the pathogen has been killed or inactivated by heat or the use of chemicals, making them incapable of replication. Also, the pathogen cannot revert to a more virulent form by mutations, as in the case of attenuated vaccines. These vaccines also provide a strong immune response and also have no danger of possible mutations. However, the killing may cause some vital information to be lost. These vaccines provide a shorter period of protection and need booster shots for continued immunity.

Examples: Polio, Hepatitis A

Toxoids

These vaccines contain the inactivated form of the toxin (called toxoid) produced by the pathogen, which is responsible for the symptoms of the disease in the human body. For example, tetanus is caused by a neurotoxin produced by the *Clostridium tetani* bacterium. So, the vaccine is prepared using a particular neurotoxin instead of the bacterium. The toxin is inactivated by heat or chemical means. These vaccines are safer. Such vaccines also require booster shots for prolonged immunity.

Examples: Diphtheria, tetanus

Subunit and Conjugate Vaccines

These vaccines use pieces of the pathogen, which are sufficient to create an immune response in the body. Subunit vaccines may contain a specific protein from a pathogen, for example, acellular pertussis vaccine and influenza vaccine (in shot form). The pneumococcal polysaccharide vaccine contains sugars from the surface of the causative bacteria. Subunit vaccines can also be prepared by recombinant technology to create viral proteins. For example, the Hepatitis B vaccine and human papillomavirus (HPV) vaccine are made by this method.

Conjugate vaccines are made using a combination of two different components, usually a piece of the pathogen and a carrier protein, which makes them more effective than subunit vaccines. For example, the pneumococcal conjugate vaccine and Haemophilus Influenza conjugate vaccine.

Vaccines of this type are safer but have a milder immune response and require adjuvants to increase their immunogenicity. Such vaccines also need booster shots to provide continued protection against diseases.

Examples: Hepatitis B vaccine and human papillomavirus (HPV) vaccine, pneumococcal conjugate vaccine and Haemophilus Influenza conjugate vaccine.

Viral Vector Vaccines

These vaccines use a modified version of a different virus as a vector to deliver information, like genetic code for the antigen, into the human body. Viruses like the influenza virus, measles virus, and adenovirus (that causes the common cold) are used as vectors. As the vector virus has been stripped of its disease-causing genes, it just acts as a vehicle for transferring the pathogen's genetic code into the human cell so that an immune response is generated for it. Such vaccines produce a strong immune response, but their manufacture is more complicated and also, and there may be some anti-vector immunity that may dampen the immune response.

Example: Vaccine against Ebola.

Messenger RNA Vaccines

mRNA vaccines consist of mRNA that encodes the required antigen and are usually delivered into the human cells enclosed in a layer of lipid nanoparticles. The mRNA gives genetic information to the recipient human cell to produce antigens for which an immune response is generated. These vaccines are safe and are now more popular. Along with generating a strong immune response, there is no risk of infection, the mRNA is easily degraded in the body, there is no anti-vector immunity, and also such vaccines are easily manufactured [5]. The main disadvantage of mRNA vaccines is their low stability which makes their storage and distribution difficult as they have to be stored at low temperatures.

DNA Vaccine

In this type of vaccine, a genetically engineered DNA sequence (plasmid) that encodes for certain proteins of the pathogen, is introduced into the human cells.

On entering the human cell, it causes the expression of the protein of the pathogen in the human cell. Consequently, antibodies are produced for this type of antigen, thereby protecting it from future infection [6]. DNA vaccines are considered to be safer than live and viral protein-based vaccines as they would pose no risk of infection and would also be easy to manufacture. They are also easy to store and transport as they are stable under room temperature conditions. At present, however, there are no approved DNA vaccines for humans, but many are under clinical studies (Table **1**).

Apart from the active ingredient, *i.e.*, the component that would cause the immune response, certain other substances are also added to vaccines to preserve and stabilize them and make them more effective. Given below is a list of ingredients added to vaccines and their roles (Table **2**) [7].

Table 1. Different types of vaccines.

Vaccine type	Examples
Live, attenuated	Measles, mumps, rubella (MMR combined vaccine) chickenpox, influenza, rotavirus
Inactivated/Killed	Polio, Hepatitis A
Toxoid (inactivated toxin)	Diphtheria, tetanus (part of DTaP combined immunization)
Subunit/conjugate	Hepatitis B vaccine, human papillomavirus (HPV) vaccine, pneumococcal conjugate vaccine and Haemophilus Influenza conjugate vaccine.
Viral vector	Vaccine against Ebola
mRNA vaccines	Cancer vaccines

Table 2. List of ingredients added to vaccines and their function.

Type of Excipient	Example(s)	Function
Preservatives	Thimerosal, ethanol, Disodium edetate dihydrate (EDTA)	To prevent contamination of the vaccine due to the growth of bacteria *etc.*, during storage
Adjuvants	Aluminium salts, CpG Adjuvant	To help enhance the body's response to the vaccine
Stabilizers	Sugars, gelatin	To keep the vaccine stable and effective after manufacture and during storage
Residual inactivating ingredients	Formaldehyde	To kill viruses or inactivate toxins during the manufacturing process
Residual antibiotics	Neomycin	To prevent contamination by bacteria during the manufacturing process
Buffers	Amines, sodium chloride, *monobasic potassium phosphate*	To maintain the pH of the vaccine

(Table 2) cont.....

Type of Excipient	Example(s)	Function
Emulsifiers	Polysorbate	To keep oil and water-containing vaccines stable

While all vaccines are well tolerated and are used only after thorough research and clinical trials, they do produce some unwanted side effects like pain and swelling at the site of administration (in case of injections), body pain, mild fever, nausea, dizziness, *etc*. This is because when a person receives a vaccine, the body identifies the antigen and innate immunity is triggered, causing white blood cells called macrophages and neutrophils to accumulate at the site. The cells start producing chemicals called cytokines. The release of cytokines leads to inflammation and pain at the site of injection. Also, in response to this stimulus, the body temperature rises slightly to curtail the replication of the antigen, causing chills and mild fever. This is a normal immune response and should not be a cause of concern and apprehension towards vaccination.

With an understanding of the function of vaccines and their types and mode of action, let us now discuss the COVID-19 vaccines in detail.

Vaccines for Protection from COVID-19

Ever since the entire world was gripped by the COVID-19 pandemic in early 2020, scientists and doctors all over began working to develop preventive and remedial strategies to counter the novel disease. The effort was highly persistent as well as collaborative, as the disease was spreading quickly all over the world, had a high mortality rate and also, no medicine was known to cure it. Doctors were treating the symptoms with the trial-and-error method, and the only protection was in its prevention, with the help of social distancing and proper sanitization. In the meantime, the virus was isolated, and its structure was studied. The major components that were identified were Nucleoproteins and viral RNA, enclosed in an envelope that comprises three structural proteins: spike protein (S), membrane protein (M) and envelope protein (E) [8].

The virus attaches itself to the receptors of host cells and enters the cell The spike glycoprotein was found to be critical for the entry of the virus inside the host cell and is, therefore, a major target for vaccine development [9]. The viral vector vaccines, for example, the Astra Zeneca vaccine and Sputnik V, are composed of an unharmful virus, like the adenovirus that causes the common cold, carrying the gene to express the spike protein. The protein subunit vaccines, such as Novavax, contain the recombinant spike protein. The inactivated virus vaccines like Covaxin and the Sinopharm vaccine do not have any genetic material, but the spike protein is intact; this disables their replication yet triggers the same immune response as the living virus. On the other hand, the RNA and DNA vaccines (*e.g.*

Pfizer and Moderna vaccines, ZyCov-D) contain genes responsible for the expression of the spike protein. On vaccination, these particles are introduced into the host's body, producing an immune response that produces antibodies. These antibodies remain in the host's body and can combat any subsequent COVID infection. The structure of SARS-CoV-2 and the different types of vaccine candidates have been shown in (Fig. **2**).

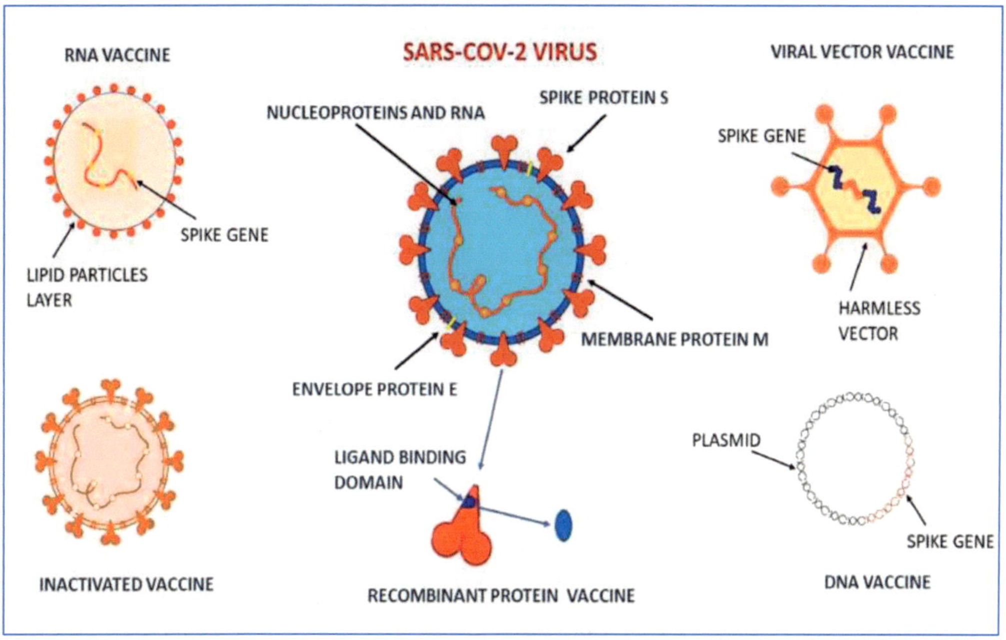

Fig. (2). Structure of the coronavirus and the different types of vaccines.

Once the gene sequence of the virus was published in January 2020, the development of a preventive COVID-19 vaccine became a top priority, with unprecedented collaboration between pharmaceutical companies and governments to accelerate the process. The development of a vaccine that would normally take several years was now being done within 1-2 years, by condensing the clinical trials. As a consequence of the continued efforts of scientists and pharmaceutical companies, as many as 8 vaccines have been approved for emergency use by WHO so far, while 140 more are in clinical development and another 194 are in pre-clinical development [10].

As of now, WHO has listed eight COVID-19 vaccines for emergency use (Table **3**). Besides these eight, several others like Sputnik V, Sinopharm WIBP, Convidicea, Sanofi–GSK and a few others are in various stages of being considered by the WHO for emergency use.

Table 3. List of vaccines approved by WHO for emergency use against COVID-19.

Name	Brand Name	Developed by	Type of Vaccine	Date of Who Approval
BNT162b2	Comirnaty	Pfizer and BioNTech	Nucleoside modified mRNA	31 December 2020
AZD1222	Covishield Vaxzervria	AstraZeneca and Oxford University	Recombinant ChAdOx1 adenoviral vector encoding the Spike protein antigen of the SARS-CoV-2	15 February 2021
Ad26.COV2.S	Janssen COVID-19 Vaccine	Johnson & Johnson-Janssen	Recombinant, replication-incompetent adenovirus type 26 (Ad26) vectored vaccine encoding the (SARS-CoV-2) Spike (S) protein	12 March 2021
mRNA-1273	Spikevax	Moderna	mRNA-based vaccine encapsulated in lipid nanoparticle (LNP)	30 April 2021
SARS-CoV-2 Vaccine	Hayat-Vax	Sinopharm-BBIBP	Inactivated, produced in Vero cells	7 May 2021
CoronaVac	CoronaVac	Sinovac Biotech	Inactivated, produced in Vero cells	1 June 2021
BBV152	Covaxin	Bharat Biotech with ICMR	Inactivated, produced in Vero cells	3 November 2021
NVX-CoV2373	Novavax	Novavax and the Coalition for Epidemic Preparedness Innovations (CEPI)	Recombinant subunit vaccine encapsulated in lipid nanoparticle	17 December 2021

The Indian Perspective

As early as September 2020, India announced that the country was planning to approve, manufacture, as well as begin distribution of a COVID-19 vaccine in early 2021 [11], beginning with the vaccination of 30 million frontline health workers who were dealing directly with COVID patients [12]. The Oxford–AstraZeneca vaccine was given emergency approval in January 2021 by the Drug Controller General of India (DCGI). This vaccine was manufactured by the Serum Institute of India under the brand name Covishield. Another vaccine that received approval was BBV152, which was given the brand name Covaxin and was developed by Bharat Biotech in association with the Indian Council of Medical Research and the National Institute of Virology [13]. Although Covaxin had not completed the requisite phase 3 clinical trials at that time, it was approved by DCGI for emergency use in places where Covishield was unavailable, due to the urgency of the pandemic situation, with the cautionary advice of 'clinical trial mode' given [14].

The process of manufacturing the two vaccines was then started, along with putting together the infrastructure for their proper storage, transport facilities and distribution; also, healthcare workers were trained to conduct the massive vaccination drive across the country. Finally, on 16th January 2021, India began its vaccination programme, with more than 3,000 vaccination centres all over the country [15]. During the initial phase of vaccination, there was a low turnout, due to concerns about the safety and efficacy of the vaccines, along with some technical problems [16]. However, around 14 million people, including healthcare workers, police and military personnel and sanitation workers, were vaccinated in the first phase of the vaccination drive [17].

In the second phase of the vaccination drive, all citizens over the age of 60, as well as those between the ages of 45 and 60 with comorbidities, were eligible for vaccination. It was during this time that the deadly second wave of the pandemic gripped India and the production of Covishield also hit some hurdles. In March 2021, after the completion of its clinical trial, DCGI allowed the restricted use of Covaxin in emergencies, in the public interest, bringing Covaxin at par with Covishield. In April, all residents over the age of 45 were deemed eligible for vaccination. By the end of April 2021, more than a hundred million vaccine doses had been administered [18]. In April, the Russian vaccine Sputnik V was approved by DCGI, for emergency use in India. This was done to expand the options and availability of vaccines across the nation, to curb the growing spread of the disease. Sputnik is now being distributed by Dr. Reddy's Laboratories.

The third phase of the vaccination drive began on 1 May 2021, with all residents of 18 years of age and above being deemed eligible for vaccination. In June 2021, the US-based pharmaceutical company Moderna's mRNA vaccine was approved by DCGI to be imported for emergency use, with the Indian pharma company Cipla Ltd. being the partner for distribution. In August 2021, US-based Johnson & Johnson's single-dose Janssen COVID-19 vaccine received emergency use approval in India. Later in the same month, emergency use approval was given to Zydus Cadila's COVID-19 vaccine, another indigenous vaccine, which is the first DNA vaccine against the coronavirus. In September 2021, the Indian government decided not to import Moderna and Pfizer vaccines as the currently in-use vaccines, Covishield and Covaxin, both being manufactured in India, were much cheaper, easily available and easy to store. With the continued and rigorous efforts of vaccine manufacturers, government agencies and healthcare providers, more than one billion vaccine doses had been administered, with almost half of the eligible Indian population having received the first dose of any of the three available vaccines in October 2021 [19a]. In November 2021, Covaxin also received WHO approval, which further boosted India's vaccination programme.

With the arrival of the Omicron variant of the virus and amid growing concern about the third wave of infections, experts have recommended giving booster shots of the vaccines to fully vaccinated persons. This would protect against new strains of the virus and also increase immunity. In India, booster doses are being given on a priority basis to the more vulnerable, including the elderly and healthcare workers, from 10th January 2022. Also, children aged 15-18 years are now eligible for a vaccination against COVID-19, and an extensive vaccination drive has been underway in the country since 3rd January 2022. The DCGI has approved Covaxin as of now for the vaccination of children: the other vaccines approved for children are Zydus Cadila's DNA vaccine and Serum Institute's Novavax vaccine, which are yet to be deployed. As of 26th January 2022, more than 1.6 billion total vaccine doses have been administered across India, with more than 66% of the population having received at least one dose (Fig. **3**) [19b].

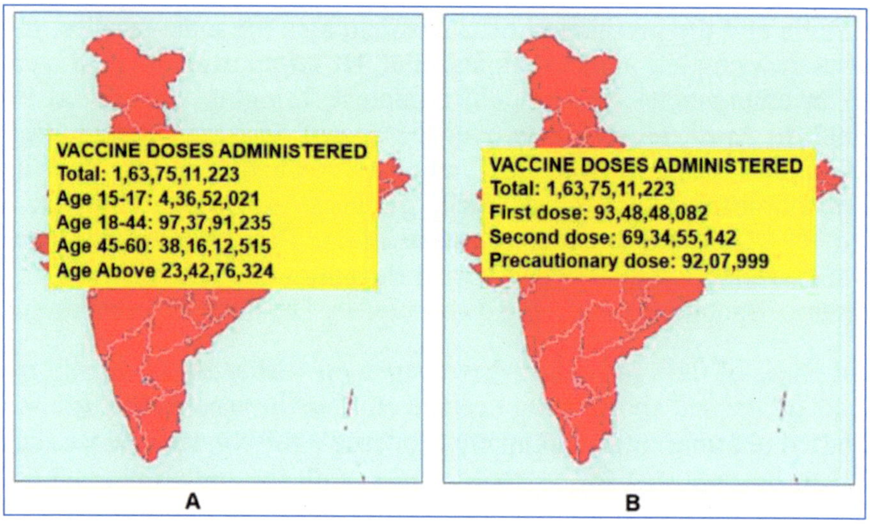

Fig. (3). A detailed account of vaccine doses administered across India. A: Age-wise account, B: Dose-wise account.

The following section delves into detail about the COVID-19 vaccines currently being used in India, as well as those in the pipeline. While three vaccines are currently in use, namely Covishield, Covaxin and Sputnik V, three more have received approval and a few more are under clinical trials. Given below is some data on vaccines against COVID-19 that are currently being used in India (Table **4**).

Table 4. COVID-19 vaccines being used in India.

Vaccine	DCGI Approval	Distribution	Doses Administered (as of January 26, 2022) [19b]
Covishield	1 January 2021	16 January 2021	More than 1.40 billion
Covaxin	3 January 2021	16 January 2021	More than 228 million
Sputnik V	12 April 2021	14 May 2021	More than 1.2 million

COVISHIELD

As mentioned earlier, Covishield has been developed by AstraZeneca and Oxford University and has been manufactured in India by the Serum Institute of India. It is a viral vector-type vaccine. The medicinal component of Covishield is ChAdOx1 nCoV-19 Corona Virus Vaccine (Recombinant), which uses an adenovirus vector derived from the chimpanzee. Some changes have been made in the genetic sequence of the vector so that its replication is prevented in human cells. The genetic sequences of SARS-CoV-2 for the transcription of spike glycoprotein have been incorporated into the vector. Each 0.5 ml dose contains 5×10^{10} viral particles (vp) [20]. The virus has then been propagated in genetically modified human embryonic kidney **HEK 293** cell lines, followed by several stages of purification to remove the cell culture [21].

Apart from the viral particles, the vaccine contains the following ingredients as well: EDTA, ethanol (preservative), L-histidine hydrochloride monohydrate, magnesium chloride hexahydrate, sodium chloride (buffers), polysorbate 80 (emulsifier), sucrose (stabilizer), and water as a solvent for injection [22].

Efficacy of Covishield

The overall efficacy of Covishield against symptomatic COVID-19 after the second dose is about 82%. It shows almost 100% efficacy in preventing the severity of the disease. Longer dose intervals within the 8 to 12 weeks range are associated with greater vaccine efficacy.

Side Effects: The vaccine is quite safe and well-tolerated, with mild to moderate side effects like injection site pain and stiffness of the arm, headache, fatigue, malaise, chills, *etc*. The side effects usually reduce within a few days; also, adverse effects are milder after the second dose.

Covaxin

BBV152, marketed under the brand name Covaxin, has been developed by Bharat Biotech, an Indian biotechnology company, in collaboration with the **Indian**

Council of Medical Research. It is an inactivated virus type of vaccine, that cannot replicate in the human body but is capable of producing an immune response. The vaccine has been developed using the Whole-Virion Inactivated Vero Cell technology. In this technique, large quantities of the virus are grown from samples of the isolated virus using vero cells. The virus is then deactivated by soaking in **beta-propiolactone**, which alters the viral proteins, making it incapable of growth. After this, Alhydroxiquim-II, an aluminium-based adjuvant, is added, which helps boost the body's response to the vaccine [23]. Apart from the inactivated virus, the vaccine contains Aluminium hydroxide gel and Imidazoquinolinone (adjuvants), 2-phenoxyethanol (preservative), and phosphate buffer saline [24].

Efficacy of Covaxin

Bharat Biotech has reported that the vaccine is 93% effective against severe COVID-19 infection. It is 64% effective against asymptomatic cases, 78% effective against symptomatic cases, and 65% effective against the Delta variant [25].

Side Effects: The side effects of Covaxin are similar to those of Covishield and include redness, swelling, pain at the injection site, fever, sweating and/ or chills, malaise, body ache, nausea and vomiting, itching and rashes, headache,*etc*.

SPUTNIK V

Sputnik V was developed by the Gamaleya National Research Centre of Epidemiology and Microbiology, which is a Russian state institute. It is being manufactured for the Indian market by Indian pharmaceutical company Panacea Biotec and is being distributed by its partner Dr. Reddy's Laboratories. Sputnik is a two-part adenovirus-based vaccine, in which the spike S-protein of coronavirus has been inserted in two different types of adenovirus vectors (rAD26 and rAD5). The two parts are administered in two doses of the vaccine. This has been done to increase the efficacy of the vaccine.

Component I of the vaccine contains recombinant adenoviral particles of the 26-serotype containing the gene for the protein S of the SARS-CoV-2 virus, in an amount of $(1.0 \pm 0.5) \times 10^{11}$ particles/dose. Apart from this active ingredient, tris (hydroxymethyl) aminomethane, sodium chloride and magnesium chloride hexahydrate (buffers), sucrose (stabilizer), EDTA sodium salt dihydrate and ethanol (preservatives), polysorbate 80 (emulsifier), water as a solvent in injection are also added.

Component II contains recombinant adenoviral particles of serotype 5 containing the gene for the protein S of the SARS-CoV-2 virus, in an amount of (1.0 ± 0.5) × 10 ^{11} particles/dose, as the active ingredient. The excipients are the same as in component I [26].

Efficacy

The efficacy of the Sputnik vaccine has been reported to be 91% by researchers, making it highly effective in the fight against COVID-19 [27].

Side Effects

The side effects are similar to those with other vaccines and include flu-like illness, headache, fatigue, injection-site pain and redness.

A comparison of the three vaccines in use in India has been given in (Fig. **4**).

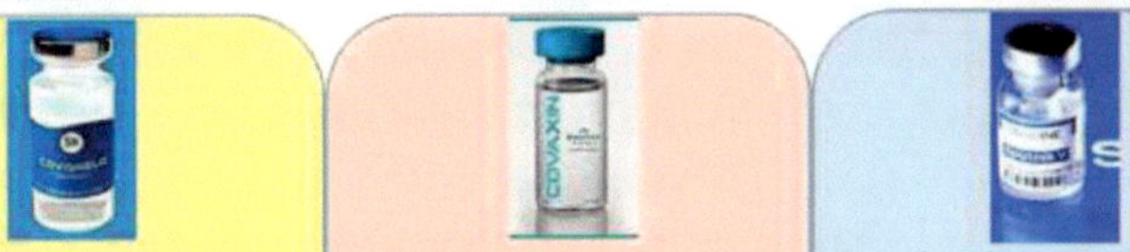

	COVISHIELD	COVAXIN	SPUTNIK V
TYPE	Viral vector type vaccine	Inactivated virus type vaccine	Viral vector type vaccine
EFFICACY	About 90%	About 81%	About 91%
DOSE INTERVAL	12-16 weeks	4-6 weeks	3 weeks
MAIN INGREDIENT	Recombinant Adenovirus inserted with SARS-CoV-2 spike protein	Inactivated virus	2 types of Recombinant Adenovirus inserted with SARS-CoV-2 spike protein
COMMON SIDE EFFECTS	Injection site pain and stiffness of arm, headache, fatigue, mild fever	Injection site swelling, pain, fever, sweating, chills, body ache, nausea	Flu-like illness, headache, fatigue, injection-site pain and redness

Fig. (4). Comparison of the three COVID-19 vaccines currently being used in India.

While the above three vaccines are currently in use in India, Cadila's indigenous vaccine ZyCoV-D, Biological E's Corbevax and Serum Institute-manufactured Covovax have received approval from DCGI and may soon be added to the immunization program.

ZyCoV-D is the world's first DNA vaccine to be approved for use against COVID-19. It contains the non-replicating plasmid containing the gene that expresses the SARS-CoV-2 spike protein [28]. The plasmid has been produced from E. coli. It has been developed by Indian pharma company Cadila Healthcare Ltd. in association with Biotechnology Industry Research Assistance Council. It uses a novel needle-free jet injector with which a fine stream of the liquid to be injected, is made to penetrate the skin and deliver the vaccine to the proper tissue. This would help to reduce the side effects associated with the injection of vaccine, such as pain, redness, swelling *etc*. The overall effectiveness of the vaccine has been reported to be 66%. ZyCoV-D is the first vaccine approved for use in India in those aged 12 years and above [29].

Corbevax is a protein subunit vaccine that has been developed by the **Texas Children's Hospital** Centre for Vaccine Development and **Baylor College of Medicine**, Texas [30]. It is being developed and manufactured by Biological E Limited, an Indian biopharmaceutical firm with funding from Coalition for Epidemic Preparedness Innovations (CEPI), and has received emergency use approval from DCGI on 28th December 2021. It contains a recombinant protein similar to the receptor-binding domain of the spike protein on the surface of SARS-CoV-2, that has been produced from *Pichia pastoris,* along with the adjuvants alhydrogel, *i.e.,* aluminium hydroxide gel, and CpG 1018 (Cytosine phosphoguanine (CpG), a synthetic form of DNA that mimics bacterial and viral genetic material) [31] that help in stimulating the immune response. Corbevax has completed two Phase III clinical trials and is safe and well-tolerated along with being immunogenic.

Covovax (also known as Novavax vaccine) is a SARS-CoV-2 recombinant spike protein vaccine (SARS-CoV-2rS) [32]. This vaccine uses part of the spike protein of the coronavirus and can be considered as a virus-like particle vaccine; however, it does not contain any genetic material and to make it non-infective, the protein is formulated as a nanoparticle. To enhance its immunogenicity, the adjuvant Matrix-M1 is used, which is a saponin prepared with cholesterol and phospholipids in the form of nanoparticles [33]. It has been developed by Novavax, USA, and is being manufactured by the Serum Institute of India. Phase three clinical trials were completed in December 2021, and the vaccine was found to be 90% effective overall [34].

Besides these, some other vaccines are currently in development stages in India, with their clinical trials going on. Among them are Bharat Biotech's intranasal vaccine BBV154, an adenoviral vector vaccine [35], and Genova Biopharmaceuticals and HDT Biotech Corporation's RNA vaccine HGC019 [36].

CONCLUSION

The combined and continuous efforts of scientists, pharmaceutical companies and also governments have resulted in the development of several vaccines against COVID-19 that have been approved by WHO for emergency use. While eight vaccines are being used worldwide to immunize people against the disease, hundreds more are in different phases of development. As a result of such an unprecedented collective response to the pandemic, more than nine billion vaccine shots have been administered worldwide [37], out of which more than one billion have been done in India. More than 50% of the world's population is now fully vaccinated, and with the development and production of more vaccines, this figure continues to rise. Even though the disease continues to wreak havoc worldwide, with the virus undergoing mutations, giving rise to novel variants, there is yet no medicine to treat it fully as of now. In such a bleak scenario, the vaccination program has brought some relief, reducing the mortality rate and severity of the disease. This has been particularly noticeable during the current Omicron wave of the infection, where fully vaccinated persons experienced much milder symptoms. The Corona-virus pandemic will only subside when a drug is developed to kill the virus upon infection; in the meantime, more people need to be vaccinated all over the world, and COVID protocol needs to be strictly followed.

CONSENT FOR PUBLICATION

Not applicable.

CONFLICT OF INTEREST

The authors declare no conflict of interest, financial or otherwise.

ACKNOWLEDGEMENTS

Declared none.

REFERENCES

[1] Brunson EK. Vaccine. https://www.britannica.com/science/vaccine

[2] Plotkin SA. Vaccines: the fourth century. Clin Vaccine Immunol 2009; 16(12): 1709-19. [http://dx.doi.org/10.1128/CVI.00290-09] [PMID: 19793898]

[3] Ehrenfeld E, Modlin J, Chumakov K. Future of polio vaccines. Expert Rev Vaccines 2009; 8(7): 899-905. [http://dx.doi.org/10.1586/erv.09.49] [PMID: 19545205]

[4] https://www.historyofvaccines.org/content/articles/different-types-vaccines

[5] Pardi N, Hogan MJ, Porter FW, Weissman D. mRNA vaccines — a new era in vaccinology. Nat Rev Drug Discov 2018; 17(4): 261-79.

[http://dx.doi.org/10.1038/nrd.2017.243] [PMID: 29326426]

[6] Liu S, Wang S, Lu S. DNA immunization as a technology platform for monoclonal antibody induction. Emerg Microbes Infect 2016; 5(1): 1-12. [http://dx.doi.org/10.1038/emi.2016.27] [PMID: 27048742]

[7] https://www.cdc.gov/vaccines/vac-gen/additives.htm

[8] Brian DA, Baric RS. Coronavirus genome structure and replication. Curr Top Microbiol Immunol 2005; 287: 1-30. [http://dx.doi.org/10.1007/3-540-26765-4_1] [PMID: 15609507]

[9] Li F, Li W, Farzan M, Harrison SC. Structure of SARS coronavirus spike receptor-binding domain complexed with receptor. Science 2005; 309(5742): 1864-8. [http://dx.doi.org/10.1126/science.1116480] [PMID: 16166518]

[10] https://www.who.int/publications/m/item/draft-landscape-of-covid-19-candidate-vaccines

[11] https://www.oneindia.com/india/expect-covid-19-vaccine-by-early-next-year-will-take-f-rst-shot-if-any-trust-deficit-vardhan-3148414.html

[12] Kaul R. 30 Million Frontline Workers To Get Covid-19 Vaccine In Phase 1. https://www.hindustantimes.com/india-news/30-million-frontline-worke-s-to-get-covid-19-vaccine-in-phase-1/story-W76e1pJ7toA4aod3hH234O.html

[13] https://www.bbc.com/news/world-asia-india-55520658?via=webuproar

[14] https://indianexpress.com/article/india/bharat-biotechs-covaxin-covid-vaccine-approval-cdsco-7130213/

[15] https://www.thehindu.com/news/national/coronavirus-worlds-largest-vaccination-programme-b-gins-in-india-on-january-16/article33582069.ece

[16] Prasad R. Vaccine dilemma- to take or not to take Covaxin. https://www.thehindu.com/sci-tech/health/vaccine-dilemma-to-take-or-not-to-take-covaxin/article33577223.ece

[17] Allana A. Opinion | How Do You Vaccinate 13 Billion People? 2021. https://www.nytimes.com/2021/03/15/opinion/india-covid-vaccine.html

[18] https://economictimes.indiatimes.com/news/india/tika-utsav-indias-covid-19-vaccination-co-erage-exceeds-11-crore-mark/articleshow/82063145.cms

[19] https://dashboard.cowin.gov.in/https://dashboard.cowin.gov.in/

[20] https://clinicaltrials.gov/ct2/show/NCT04400838

[21] https://www.ema.europa.eu/en/documents/covid-19-vaccine-safety-update/covid-19-vaccine-safety-update-vaxzevria-previously-covid-19-vaccine-astrazeneca-14-april-2021_en.pdf

[22] https://www.seruminstitute.com/pdf/covishield_fact_sheet.pdf

[23] Corum J, Zimmer C. How Bharat Biotech's Vaccine Works. https://www.nytimes.com/interactive/2021/health/bharat-biotech-covid-19-vaccine.html

[24] https://www.fda.gov.ph/wp-content/uploads/2021/04/COVAXIN-Product-Info.pdf

[25] Ella R, Vadrevu KM, Jogdand H, *et al.* Safety and immunogenicity of an inactivated SARS-CoV-2 vaccine, BBV152: a double-blind, randomised, phase 1 trial. Lancet Infect Dis 2021; 21(5): 637-46. [http://dx.doi.org/10.1016/S1473-3099(20)30942-7] [PMID: 33485468]

[26] Gam-COVID-Wack, Medum.ru: [cited: 30 October 2021]. Available from: https://medum.ru/sputnik-v

[27] Logunov DY, Dolzhikova IV, Shcheblyakov DV, *et al.* Safety and efficacy of an rAd26 and rAd5 vector-based heterologous prime-boost COVID-19 vaccine: an interim analysis of a randomised controlled phase 3 trial in Russia. Lancet 2021; 397(10275): 671-81. [http://dx.doi.org/10.1016/S0140-6736(21)00234-8] [PMID: 33545094]

[28] Dey A, Chozhavel Rajanathan TM, Chandra H, *et al.* Immunogenic potential of DNA vaccine candidate, ZyCoV-D against SARS-CoV-2 in animal models. Vaccine 2021; 39(30): 4108-16. [http://dx.doi.org/10.1016/j.vaccine.2021.05.098] [PMID: 34120764]

[29] Kaul R. Covid vaccine for children in India by September, says ICMR-NIV director. Hindustan Times. 18 August 2021.

[30] Biological E. 2021. https://www.clinicaltrialsarena.com/news/biological-e-vaccine-trial/

[31] Campbell JD. Development of the CpG Adjuvant 1018: A Case Study. Methods Mol Biol 2017; 1494: 15-27. [http://dx.doi.org/10.1007/978-1-4939-6445-1_2] [PMID: 27718183]

[32] https://www.ema.europa.eu/en/news/ema-starts-rolling-review-novavaxs-covid-19-vac-ine-nvx-cov2373

[33] Rajput ZI, Hu S, Xiao C, Arijo AG. Adjuvant effects of saponins on animal immune responses. J Zhejiang Univ Sci B 2007; 8(3): 153-61. [http://dx.doi.org/10.1631/jzus.2007.B0153] [PMID: 17323426]

[34] Dunkle Lisa M, *et al.* Efficacy and Safety of NVX-CoV2373 in Adults in the United States and Mexico. N Engl J Med 2021; NEJMoa2116185.

[35] Hassan AO, Kafai NM, Dmitriev IP, *et al.* A Single-Dose Intranasal ChAd Vaccine Protects Upper and Lower Respiratory Tracts against SARS-CoV-2. Cell 2020; 183(1): 169-184.e13. [http://dx.doi.org/10.1016/j.cell.2020.08.026] [PMID: 32931734]

[36] mRNA Based Vaccines – HGC019". Gennova Biopharmaceuticals Limited. [cited: 30 October 2021]. Available from: https://gennova.bio/mrna-vaccines/

[37] Covid vaccines: How fast is progress around the world?. https://www.bbc.com/news/world-56237778

CHAPTER 8

COVID-19 Vaccination Acceptance, Management and Concerns: A Survey-Based Study

Saima Arif[1,*], **Ayushi Tewari**[2], **Tuba Siddiqui**[3] and **Sumaiyya Khan**[4]

[1] *Toxicokinetics Laboratory, CSIR- Indian Institute of Toxicology Research (IITR), Lucknow-226001, Uttar Pradesh, India*

[2] *Department of Education, District Institute of Education and Training (DIET), Lucknow-226007, Uttar Pradesh, India*

[3] *Department of Biochemistry, Integral Institute of Medical Sciences and Research, Lucknow-226026, Uttar Pradesh, India*

[4] *Department of Food & Nutrition, Era University, Lucknow-226003, Uttar Pradesh, India*

Abstract: The COVID-19 pandemic has had a significant impact, especially in the last 2 years, and inflicted a grave loss globally. The world came together to devise various protocols and preventive measures to battle this viral outbreak. The chapter explores the various immediate medicinal measures to cure COVID infections. The Government of India initiated the process of vaccine manufacture and distribution among the population. This was met by various hurdles, namely myths, misconceptions, misinformation and concerns regarding the vaccines and the disease itself. This was majorly reported in the rural regions of India where the vaccination was not successful in the desired results; this might have been due to various reasons, such as lack of awareness among the rural population or due to the difficulty faced in the transportation and storage of Corona vaccines. This chapter attempts to shed light on the acceptance of the COVID-19 vaccines by the Indian population and also discusses the same concerning the rural population and proposes plans to expedite the Corona Vaccines to such areas. The Government of India initiated a Co-WIN vaccine delivery management system to encourage people and create awareness to fight against this pandemic by opting for vaccination. An independent survey was conducted that consisted of a questionnaire addressing acceptance, management and concerns about the COVID-19 vaccination. Among 211 respondents, 19.6% (41 respondents) were either doctors or medical professionals. The survey provided insight into vaccine awareness among frontline workers and the general public of India.

Keywords: Coronavirus, COVID-19, India, Medicinal Measures, Misconceptions, Rural, Vaccination, Vaccine Management.

* **Corresponding author Saima Arif**: Toxicokinetics Laboratory, CSIR- Indian Institute of Toxicology Research (IITR), Lucknow-226001, Uttar Pradesh, India: E-mail: saimarif305@gmail.com

Alfred J. Lawrence & Tahmeena Khan (Eds.)

INTRODUCTION

The novel beta-coronavirus SARS-CoV-2 is thought to have originated from bats in Wuhan, China last year in 2019. Crossing the species barrier, it entered human beings with the furtherance of infection through human-to-human transmission. The beta-coronaviruses have caused three zoonotic outbreaks, namely, SARS-CoV (2002-03), MERS-CoV (2012) and SARS-CoV-2 (2019- till date) in the last 2 decades [1]. Despite the greatest efforts of governments and the World Health Organization (WHO), the virus has spread to 188 nations and 25 territories across the world due to the virus's tremendous transmission capacity [2]. Those with any other co-morbid diseases are more likely to become infected and experience severe symptoms. The virus is believed to have a 5.1-day incubation period. Fever, dry cough, shortness of breath, chills and diarrhoea are some of the symptoms of the disease [3]. Coronaviruses are pleomorphic and have strange projections of S protein protruding from their surface. The genome of the new coronavirus is translated into a polyprotein, which is then processed into 16 non-structural proteins (NSPs) [4]. The non-structural proteins aid in genome replication, capping, and tailing, all of which are required for viral maintenance [5]. The SARS-CoV-2 virus also has four structural proteins encoded by the 3'end of the viral genome: spike (S), nucleocapsid (N), envelope (E), and membrane (M) [6]. The S glycoprotein, a multi-functional trans-membrane protein, is one of the four structural proteins that play an essential role in viral attachment and entry into the host cell [6]. The S protein is made up of two subunits, S1 and S2, that divide into distinct functional domains. The N-terminal domain (NTD) and the Receptor Binding Domain (RBD), both of which include a conserved receptor-binding motif (RBM), make up the S1 subunit [7]. COVID-19 vaccinations are often designed to produce S protein-neutralising antibodies. According to studies, there is practically no cross-neutralization between SARS-CoV and SARS-CoV-2 sera, indicating that people who have recovered from one illness are not immune to the other. More than 5,000 full-length genomes of SARS-CoV-2 have been obtained from various countries, defining the polymorphism in S and other viral proteins that are important for vaccine development. S protein has been used in the majority of COVID-19 vaccines produced [8]. The global effort to develop a COVID-19 vaccination that is both safe and effective is bearing fruit. Around the world, almost two dozen vaccines have been approved, with many more in work. As of 29th October 2021, a total of seven vaccines have been approved to use in India, and 13 vaccines are still under trial [9].

Medicinal Solution for Treatment of COVID-19 Disease

As the study of various aspects of the virus that causes COVID-19 disease was yet to be done for the development of effective medicine, seeing the speed of spread of infection and the number of fatalities it was causing, there was the need for urgent treatment of the disease. For this, Allopathic, Unani and homeopathic treatment approaches were made.

Among Allopathic approaches was the use of oxygen therapy, intravenous fluid infusion with life support in dangerous cases, antiviral combination with antibiotic, convalescent plasma therapy, anti-fungal treatment and extracorporeal membrane oxygenation (ECMO) [10]. Researchers also evaluated that the already existing anti-viral medicines such as penciclovir, ribavirin, nitazoxanide, remdesivir (GS-5734), nafamostat, favipiravir (T-750) or Avigan, avermectins, dexamethasone, EIDD-2801, hydroxychloroquine, chloroquine, and convalescent plasma (CP) therapy were effective against the infection of SARS-CoV-2 [11].

The Unani and Ayurvedic treatments, which are on plant-based medicine, were also utilized for the treatment as parts of many plants are known to be effective against the various viral strains. Their decoction is used in treatment. Homeopathic treatments involved the use of Arsenic Album 30 for the treatment, though there was no clinical evidence for this medicine to be effective. As it was also seen that the deaths were more among the older person than young, it was suggested to use immune system boosters to prevent the spread of infection [12].

Development of COVID-19 Vaccine

Major biotech firms, namely, the Serum Institute of India, Bharat Biotech, Premas Biotech, and Zydus Cadila, have been engaged actively in the vaccine creation for COVID-19 disease. The Serum Institute of India collaborated with Codagenix, a major US pharmaceutical, and produced the Covishield vaccine, and other Indian institutes also collaborated with Oxford University for the production of the Oxford vaccine or ChAdOx1 nCoV-19 [13].

The Bharat Biotech, in collaboration with the Indian Council of Medical Research-National Institute of Virology, developed COVAXIN, India's indigenous vaccine. The Bharat Biotech, in partnership with Thomas Jefferson University, also entered the animal trial. Premas Biotech used a recombinant proteins development platform to develop the new vaccine against COVID-19 jointly with Akers Biosciences [14].

MATERIAL AND METHODS

The study was conducted between 16th September - 23rd September 2021, using an online questionnaire-based survey named "A survey on potential acceptance, management, and concerns related to COVID-19 Vaccines in India", comprising 34 questions in total. The google form was divided into two sections; the first section was concerned with the mandatory questions such as gender, profession, age group, whether or not received COVID vaccine, and other related details to the vaccination. The second section comprised questions that were majorly related to the concerns and health effects of the vaccines. The study was carried out following the Helsinki Declaration's guidelines. A questionnaire survey offers a practical and inexpensive way to gather data from the targeted respondents. This survey-based research method was adopted to provide a broad capability, such that a more accurate sample can be ensured to gather the result. This would help in drawing conclusions and making important decisions. In this survey, a total of 211 responses were recorded, of which 19.6% of respondents were either medical professionals or doctors. The survey catered to the purpose of providing a peek into vaccine awareness among the Indian population, majorly frontline workers and the general public of India.

ACCEPTANCE OF COVID-19 VACCINE IN INDIA

Vaccine Hesitancy

Vaccines are believed to be the most awaited intervention, and hundreds of research and development institutions work on it. Since the vaccine against COVID-19 was brought in for administration in such a short period, the general population has been unable to accept the fact that it can be effective and safe. Vaccine hesitancy has always been the leading concern of all time [15].

In developing countries like India, vaccine hesitancy and reluctance to accept vaccines have always existed in significant numbers, even for routine immunization. Therefore, vaccine hesitancy associated with COVID-19 vaccines is not unexpected. The overall vaccine hesitancy to routine childhood vaccines in Tamil Nadu showed a rising trend even before the COVID-19 pandemic. There were several instances of hesitancy related to the Measles-Rubella vaccine when it was introduced in campaign mode in the state in 2016. Consecutive National Family Health Surveys have shown a declining trend of vaccine coverage in Tamil Nadu despite a high performance in all other healthcare indicators [16]. A significant proportion of India belongs to the rural society and lacks in many ways, including education and digital facilities. Interestingly in India, the urban population that was highly educated and full-time employed was more likely to be hesitant to the COVID-19 vaccine. Studies show that these populations were not affected heavily due to the disruption caused by the pandemic and therefore were not that much concerned about getting vaccinated [17].

India launched the world's largest COVID-19 vaccination program on January 16th, 2021 to vaccinate its 900 million eligible population. During phase 1, around 30 million healthcare and frontline workers were to be vaccinated, followed by the elderly and those with co-morbidities, people in the age group of 45-60 and 18-44 in the subsequent phases at the beginning of May 2021. Though the vaccination drive in India faced various logistical hiccups, India managed to surpass the USA in administering the maximum number of doses in the world [18].

According to WHO, vaccine hesitancy can be defined as “delay in acceptance or refusal of vaccination despite the availability of vaccination services”. WHO recognized vaccine hesitancy as one of the 10 leading threats to global health [18]. Some of the various reasons that were discussed for the non-acceptance of vaccines included concerns regarding the vaccine’s safety and effectiveness, side effects(negative), a lack of confidence in the health system, misconceptions about the vaccines, and a lack of community awareness about the diseases that can be prevented through vaccines. Vaccine hesitancy affects not only the person who refuses to take the vaccine but also the entire population. In India, the fake information and misguided hesitancy about the vaccines have been a substantial threat to the elimination of the pandemic and achieving herd immunity against the infection. According to our survey, in which 211 people participated, 12 respondents did not want to get vaccinated at all, the reason being the difficulty in accepting vaccines due to misinformation and misconceptions.

Hesitancy in Rural India

Sixty-five percent of India’s population resides in rural areas, while only 33 per cent of the health infrastructure caters to their needs. People in rural India do not easily trust the treatment offered by allopathic doctors and advanced healthcare facilities, owing to cultural backwardness and anecdotal evidence. As many got infected, they chose to visit *Nadi babas* or quacks for their treatment. Many even hid their symptoms from others to avoid consulting doctors and facing the stigma that comes with the COVID-19 infection. Despite numerous sessions, dissemination of information in regional languages, and Q&A sessions, the majority of village residents are unconvinced that vaccination could protect them from the virus. Apart from this, there was a problem with the rollout itself. Vaccines could not be stored by the authorities at the right temperature as facilities to do so often do not exist in rural areas. It is important to keep the dialogue with rural communities alive and provide them with the right information. To be able to do so, grassroots-level organizations need resources to be able to help vulnerable communities. It is important for frontline workers, both medical and social workers, to feel supported and acknowledged. A healthy discourse on rural communities in the media will go a long way. Above all, it is important to reassure them to get proper medical treatment. The government, as well as non-profit organisations (NGOs), should support them to provide necessary equipment and resources and assure them that they will not be left alone in this apocalypse [19].

Plan to Expedite Vaccination in Rural India

The rural population (% of the total population) in India was reported at 65.074% in 2020 [20]. In a country where more than half of the population constitutes the rural sector, it is obvious that extra measures must be taken to expedite the COVID-19 vaccination to in rural regions. A few concerns arise when rural regions and their population are mentioned. The major concerns which were related to the vaccination drive could be listed as follows:

1. Many rural areas are inaccessible and isolated. Such areas are usually away from basic medical and healthcare amenities.

2. The population is not very literate or educated, and thus, is not much aware of the vaccination schemes. This hinders the process of vaccination to a great degree.

To vaccinate the population against poliovirus, the Indian government and medical authorities run and established various camps and vaccination posts. Similar measures could be taken with regard to the rural population to vaccinate them against coronavirus too.

Socio-Demographic Variables Affecting Vaccine Acceptance

Delaying acceptance or refusing vaccines against COVID-19 despite the fact that their availability has become a primary obstacle in achieving the required goal of vaccinating the maximum population in India. The rise in the number of cases in India during the second wave was devastating and affected both the mental health and economic status of the people regardless of their social status, gender, and age. Even though vaccine against COVID-19 has been made available in both private and government organizations, there is still a considerate population not willing to get vaccinated for several reasons. The residents of the rural area were under the influence of misconceptions like infertility issues in men and women; the aged population was worried that they might have harmful side effects because of their co-morbidities, people with lower economic status didn't want to get the vaccine because they were afraid that they would have to pay for the vaccine [21].

Beliefs and Barriers Associated with Vaccination among the General Public

Vaccine hesitancy among the general population was induced due to several concerns. According to our survey, 53.1% of respondents (Out of 211 respondents) (Fig. (**1**)) didn't have any concerns regarding the vaccination, but other respondents were worried about the effectiveness of the vaccine. Few hesitated because they thought that the vaccination may cause harmful side effects. People also believe that once they come in contact with COVID-19, they don't have to get the vaccine because they are already immune to it. Pregnancy, CRP (C- reactive protein) less than 30, diabetes, obesity, *etc.*, also act as barriers. Apart from these reasons, some respondents did want to get vaccinated but had a problem reaching the vaccination centres or were confused about which vaccine they should get because of the availability of more than one vaccine in India.

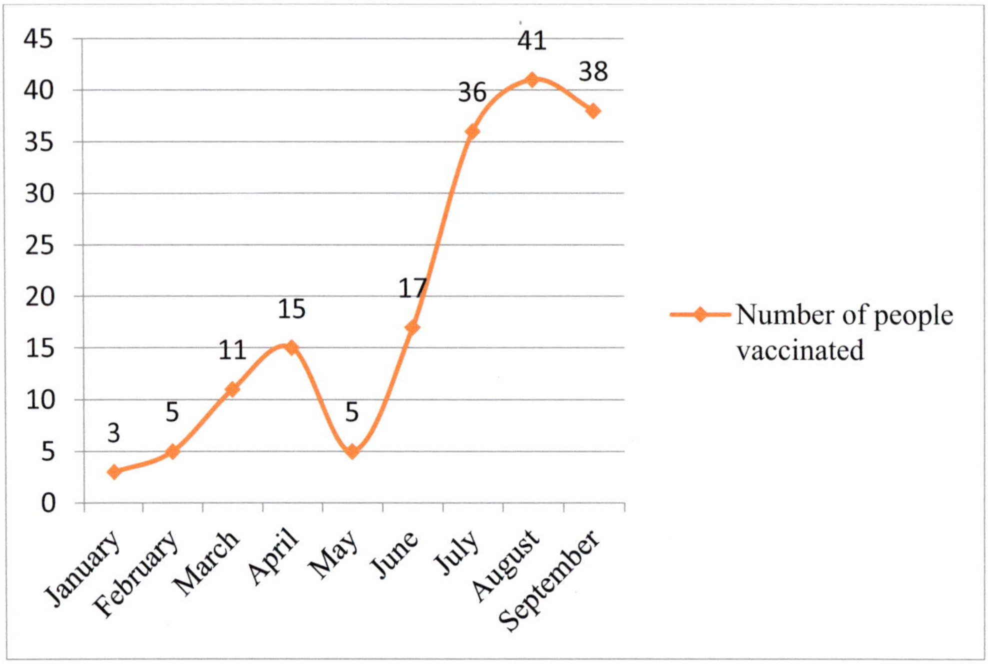

Fig. (1). Chart showing the trend in Indian population vaccination (case study).

Factors Affecting Vaccine Acceptance in India

The effort of vaccination is also facing resistance because of the myths surrounding it-

1. COVID-19 vaccines are dangerous because they are untested.

2. Coronavirus vaccines can cause infertility issues in men and women.

3. It will alter a person's DNA.

However, these myths have been busted with satisfactory explanations, as discussed ahead [22].

Myth 1: COVID-19 Vaccines are Dangerous and Untested

Many people doubt that COVID-19 vaccines are unsafe because they were developed in record time and may not have undergone the safety tests for human administration. However, this is far from the truth because all the Government-authorized vaccines under the legal labels are completely safe. All the vaccines, such as Covishield, Covaxin, Moderna, or any other authorized vaccine, are completely safe for human administration as no step of trial has been skipped before authorizing it for public use (Fig. **2**).

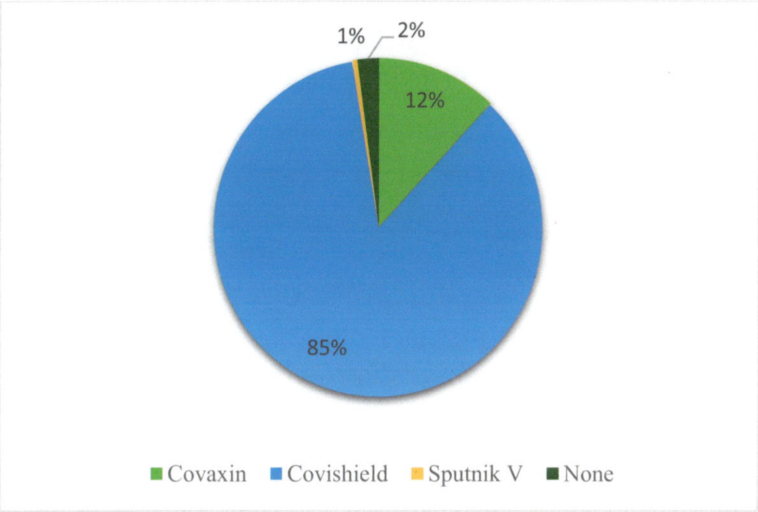

Fig. (2). A case study of the vaccines favoured in India.

Myth 2: Coronavirus Vaccines can Cause Infertility Issues in Men and Women

This is another widespread myth that the vaccines against COVID-19 will render a person infertile. There are posts and blogs on the internet that suggest that COVID vaccines can destroy the placenta proteins in females leading to their infertility, there are similar baseless claims that have been made regarding male reproductive health too. These claims are completely false.

Myth 3: Coronavirus Vaccines can Alter the Receiver's DNA

This rumour was spread in India that injecting the COVID-19 vaccine can alter an individual's DNA because of the mRNA component of the vaccine. However, the fact is completely in contrast to the myth. The fact is that the mRNA component of the vaccine instructs the body's immune system to synthesize 'spike protein' since it is the essential component of Coronavirus. Our immune system will memorize the spike protein and trigger the appropriate immune response when it detects the COVID virus in our body.

Strategies to Improve Vaccination Acceptance

The fact that the general population starts accepting newly developed vaccines without hesitancy depends upon how much knowledge about the vaccine they have. The accelerated development of the vaccine contributed to the rise in a negative attitude towards the vaccine among the general public. There are several ways to solve these issues and improve vaccine acceptance [15].

• Develop reliable media sources to make people aware of the benefits and availability of vaccines. Knowing that the vaccine is beneficial will be a plus factor in the acceptance of the vaccine.

• Health workers should be supported in their decision to take vaccine shots so that they might build up confidence and can further recommend their patients to get vaccinated. A doctor's recommendation can help clear doubts and misinformation related to the COVID vaccine.

• Educational campaigns should be promoted for those who are in the higher risk category of rejecting vaccines and for those who are under the influence of misconceptions.

• The government authorities should take initiatives through social media and attenuate concerns regarding the safety and efficacy of the vaccine by providing the right information. They should try and resolve the false beliefs that are causing hindrances in vaccinating people. They can also provide appropriate knowledge about the vaccine, which might increase people's trust and encourage them to get vaccine shots.

• Further studies on the safety and efficacy of the COVID-19 vaccine should be made available on the web so that people can access it easily and satisfy their doubts. People should get their answers for why they must get vaccinated.

• Studies should be done to understand the factors that encourage vaccine hesitancy so that policymakers can bring up more efficient strategies to implement public vaccination drives.

MANAGEMENT OF COVID-19 VACCINATION IN INDIA

The Government of India initiated its vaccination drive on the 16th of January 2021. But this event itself was preceded by an intricate plan of management which came to be known as Co-WIN ("winning over COVID-19"). Co-WIN vaccine delivery management system was a well-thought-out plan made with the motive to vaccinate the Indian population and thus, fight the COVID-19 pandemic. According to the Ministry of Health and Welfare (MOHW), "*India's National COVID-19 Vaccination Strategy is predicated on scientific and epidemiological evidence and focuses on systematic end-to-end planning. This strategy derives guidance from Global Best Practices, SoPs of WHO also as recommendations of India's foremost experts within the National Expert Group on Vaccine Administration for COVID-19 (NEGVAC)*" [23]. Fig. (**3**) shows how India's vaccination drive was supposed to work out (Source: The Hindustan Times).

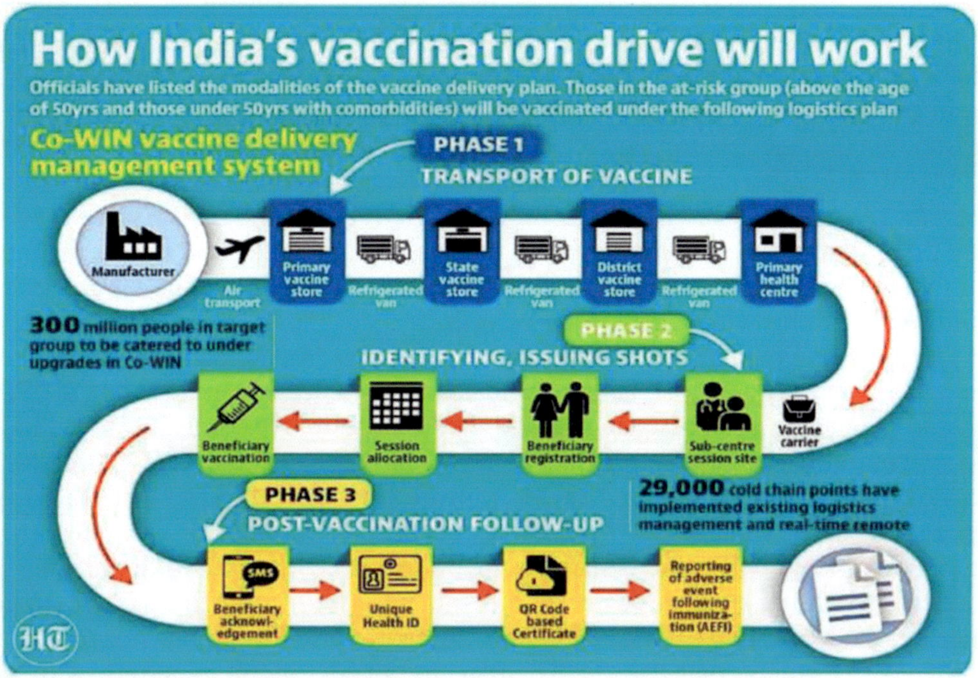

Fig. (3). Co-WIN vaccine delivery management system (Courtesy: The Hindustan Times).

According to this management system, the vaccination process was divided into phases ranging from phase 1 to phase 3. The flowchart clearly shows the process of handling and management of vaccines. Phase 1 focused on the transport of the vaccine from the manufacturer to the primary health centre, passing through the primary vaccine store, state vaccine store, and district vaccine store. Phase 2 dealt with identifying and issuing shots to individuals for the sole purpose of beneficiary vaccination, while Phase 3 dealt with the post-vaccination follow-up.

Apps like Aarogya Setu and the Co-WIN website maintain an in-depth record of the progress of COVID-19 and the vaccination drive in India. Before the commencement of the vaccination drive, the Drugs Controller General of India (DCGI) had approved the emergency use of "Covishield" (Oxford-AstraZeneca formulation) followed by the authorization of interim emergency use of BBV152 ("Covaxin"). By 1st March 2021, only 14 million healthcare and frontline workers could get vaccinated (the original target being 30 million), thus falling short [24]. Nonetheless, the online registration began in March. Later in the month, Covaxin concluded its trial and was issued a standard emergency use authorization. All the residents aged above 45 years were made eligible at the start of April 2021, and in the following week, Prime Minister Narendra Modi called for "*Teeka Utsav*" (vaccine festival), which was to be held from 11th to 14th April 2021. By the end of the festival, India had reached a milestone of 111 million vaccine doses [25]. This was followed by the approval of Russia's Sputnik V vaccine for emergency use in India. Phase 3 vaccination validated all the citizens aged above 18 years to register for the vaccination, and this phase commenced on the 1st of May 2021. 28th April 2021, the day phase 3 registration began, marked another milestone, wherein 13.3 million people registered, a single-day record [26]. By the start of May 2021, the initial shipment of 1,50,000 Sputnik V doses had arrived in India and two weeks later, its administration had begun. Meanwhile, phase 2 and phase 3 trials of Covaxin were approved on children aged 2 to 18 years. Up until mid-May, only online registrations for vaccination were available, but later on, walk-in registrations were allowed. The e-certificates were generated in the Aarogya Setu app and could also be accessed on the Co-WIN website. By the end of May, India had successfully administered 200 million vaccine doses in total [27]. In late June, the vaccination system reverted to centralized procurement, according to which the centre will procure up to 75% of the country's vaccine supplies from manufacturers in bulk and distribute them to states at no additional charge. Vaccines would be offered at no charge for those within the 18–44 age group. Later on, the Moderna vaccine, which was to be imported by Cipla, was approved by DCGI for emergency use. DCGI also approved the emergency use of the Johnson and Johnson single-dose vaccine in early August. Amidst all this, India had crossed a milestone of 500 million doses within six months from the onset of the vaccination program [28]. India also approved the world's first DNA-based COVID-19 vaccine Zy-CoV-D, for adults and youngsters aged 12 years and above (for emergency use). All these events related to the management of vaccination are listed in Fig. (**4**).

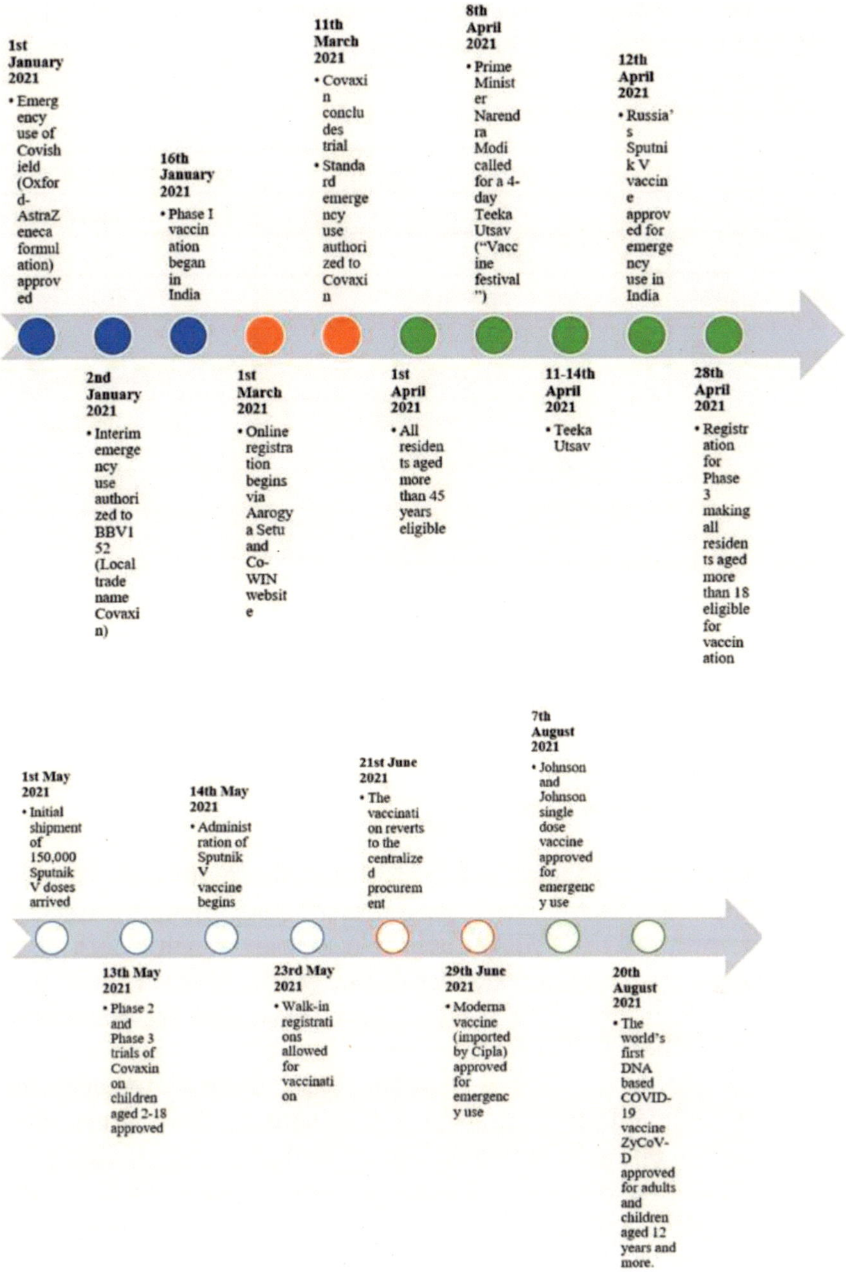

Fig. (4). Timeline of vaccine management in India.

At present, 7 vaccines have gotten approval, namely, Zy-CoV-D, mRNA-1273, Sputnik-V, Ad26.COV2.S, AZD1222, Covishield (Oxford-Astra Zeneca formulation), and Covaxin, details of which are summarized in Table **1**. Currently, 13 vaccines are undergoing trial in India [9].

Table 1. List of vaccines approved in India.

Vaccine Type	Brand Name	Manufacturing Institute/Company
DNA	Zy-CoV-D	Zydus Cadila
RNA	mRNA-1273	Moderna
Non-replicating viral vector	Sputnik V	Gamaleya
	Ad26.COV2.S	Janssen (Johnson & Johnson)
	AZD1222	Oxford/AstraZeneca
	Covishield (Oxford/AstraZeneca formulation)	Serum Institute of India
	Covaxin	Bharat Biotech

According to our survey, we found that out of 189 individuals, 83.7% had opted for vaccination from government centres, and 14.7% had opted for a private vaccination centre. We asked them the reason for opting for paid vaccines over free vaccines, to which 50.7% of responses pointed out that vaccination was paid provided by the state government. 9.9% of people could not register for government policy, and 15.5% of people found it convenient to visit a private centre. In many cases, the people went for their organization camps because employer reimbursement was available.

Many institutions and companies had made it mandatory for their employers to be fully vaccinated. The Tamil Nadu government had announced that it was a mandate for employees as well as their relations to acquire both doses of the COVID-19 vaccine to access workplaces or industries. This was done to minimize the risk of getting infected since studies have shown that vaccinated individuals have a lesser risk of being COVID-19-affected than unvaccinated ones. According to Hindustan Times, as of 13th September 2021, three states and three union territories have achieved 100% first-dose vaccination. These states and UTs are Dadra & Nagar Haveli and Daman & Diu (6.26 Lakh doses), Goa (11.83 Lakh doses), Himachal Pradesh (55.74 Lakh doses), Ladakh (1.97 Lakh doses), Lakshadweep (53,499 doses), and Sikkim (5.10 Lakh doses) [29]. It is noteworthy that as many as 25 million people got vaccinated on 17th September 2021, on the occasion of Prime Minister Narendra Modi's birthday, which became the highest single-day vaccination record in the whole world [30].

CONCERNS AMONG PEOPLE RELATED TO COVID-19 VACCINATION

Since the breakout of coronavirus disease, it is believed that despite all the measures taken to check the spread of infection, a vaccine would be the most effective tool in curbing the disease spread and bringing back normal circumstances again. The vaccines were first disseminated among medical professionals and frontline workers and then covered a large section of the population above 18 years of age. Though the successful development of vaccine and distribution programs started by the government, the acceptance of the vaccine by common people faced many challenges as well. The barriers were the concerns and misconceptions which developed among them. One of the reasons for doubt was vaccines for SARS-COV-2 virus disease developed in a short time as compared to the time taken in the development of other vaccines, this led to many concerns among people regarding its safety which also resulted in slow acceptance of it. Most of the concerns were the health problems that will/may occur after receiving the vaccination shot. The anxiety aroused as there were some unfortunate incidents cited in some people after they received either their 1st or 2nd dose of vaccination. Though the researchers on such cases later found out that the real cause of their anaphylactic shock/hyper reaction was the individual underlying health conditions such as chronic disease, lung disease, *etc.*, still these episodes stirred up many concerns about the safety of COVID-19 vaccination in a lot of minds. In some rare cases, the individuals developed a new disease after being vaccinated, for example, The Times of India (TOI) reported cases in which the blood glucose levels were altered in diabetic patients, who have maintained their sugar levels to normal through a proper diet and medication before getting the vaccine. Even the glucose level of a non-diabetic, in a 64-year-old man was found to be altered after receiving the COVID vaccination. The rise in blood pressure after getting the vaccine shot was also reported by the Times of India [31]. There have been known concerns among pregnant women about the safety of the vaccine for them.

We did an online study to explore the feelings of people about the COVID vaccine, the web-based study consisted of 32 questions about different aspects of COVID-19 vaccination including concerns and misconceptions related to it among the population. In Fig. (**5**) (this figure is drawn based on survey results) different types of concerns related to the vaccine can be noted, though about 50% (of 211 respondents) didn't have any concerns regarding the safety of the vaccine, the rest were having so many doubts.

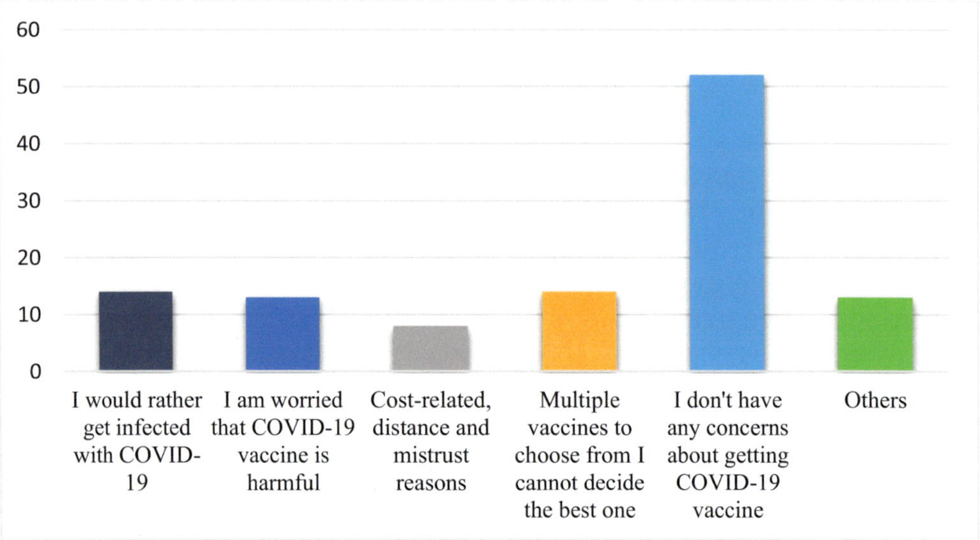

Fig. (5). Concerns regarding vaccines (Case study).

Out of the 211 respondents to the survey, 124 felt that they were not in a high-risk category to catch the viral disease, 48 people replied with 'yes' that they are in a high-risk category to contract infection according to the conditions that were put up in the questionnaire, 26 people were not sure about being in a high-risk category or not. Through this, we can roughly state that 22% of the Indian population is in a high-risk category for catching COVID-19 disease. Healthcare workers mostly were the ones who categorized themselves to be in a high-risk category to catch the disease, others were those who have low immunity, chronic disease patients, diabetics, lung infection patients, senior citizens, *etc.*

Side effects like fever, headache, and pain are common with any vaccination. But some people, due to their underlying health condition or low immunity, experience some severe side effects or even death, these incidents create major concerns among others planning to get vaccinated. Our survey graph Fig. (**6**) displays different side effects suffered by people after vaccination. It can be estimated from the figure that the common symptoms were fever, fatigue, pain, *etc.* and the severe symptoms like breathing difficulty, vomiting, rashes, *etc.*, were experienced by fewer sections. There were even 37 respondents who did not experience any side effects at all. Hence, it can be concluded that the severe side effects after vaccination aren't directly due to the vaccine dose but the underlying health condition of individuals, which is the reason for severe symptoms.

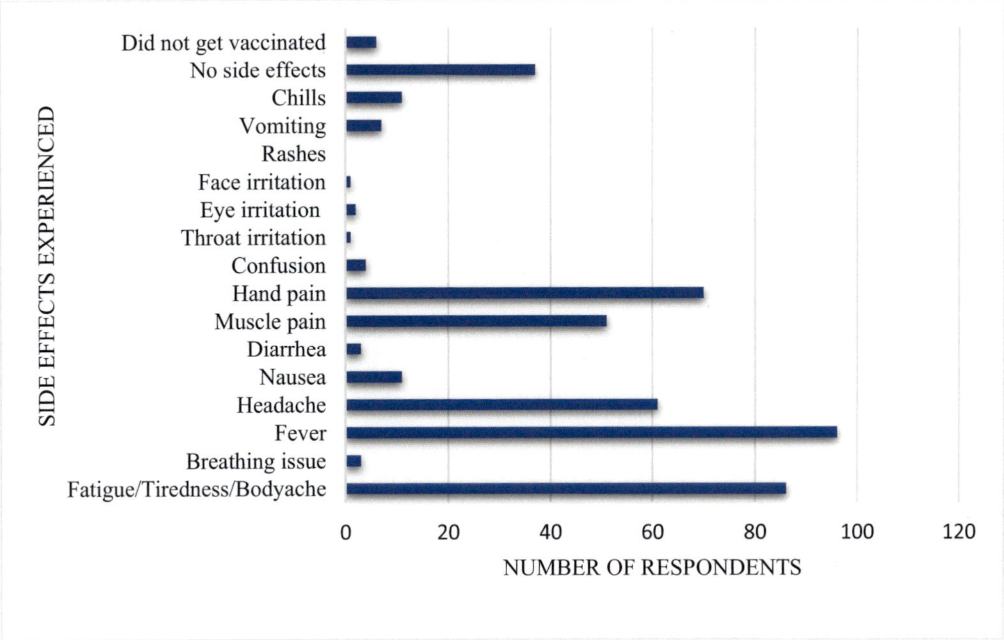

Fig. (6). Side effects faced post-vaccination.

The side effects appeared immediately in 15% of 175 people, while 82.3% didn't experience any side effects at all and 2.9% of people showed uncertainty about their experience of side effects. As estimated by the survey, 10 among the ones who didn't experience any side effects after vaccination believed that no side effect means the vaccine isn't working.

Most people (97 out of 181) relied on pain relievers like ibuprofen or paracetamol to avoid discomfort. 36 respondents showed concern that the natural antibodies might get destroyed by the vaccine.

Misconceptions/Myths Among the Indian Population About the COVID-19 Vaccine

The vaccine dissemination process did not only face challenges from concerns of people regarding the safety of vaccines but also many prevailing myths and misconceptions about it. Our country is very large in terms of population, and with too many people comes too many challenges; it becomes difficult to disperse messages to the whole population about the safety and benefits of the vaccine. The government has faced and is still facing these challenges, which stand like a wall in the acceptance of the vaccine.

From Fig. (**5**) , we can study the prevailing myths about COVID-19 vaccination among the population, which are:

- A vaccine can cause severe side effects, such as an allergic reaction.
- People who were diagnosed with COVID-19 felt that they didn't need to get vaccinated.
- Some of them didn't even plan to get vaccinated because they believed that even after getting a vaccine shot, they may contract the disease.
- The prevailing misconception is that vaccines aren't safe for pregnant women.
- Vaccines aren't tested thoroughly and might be unsafe.

Other studies also showed different myths in people's minds [22], such as:-

- The rumour is that vaccine jab causes infertility in both men and women.
- DNA can get affected by vaccination.
- The SARS-CoV-2 vaccine contains a tracking device
- COVID-19 vaccine can itself cause coronavirus disease.
- Some believed that they will test positive for coronavirus after getting vaccinated with the COVID-19 vaccine.
- The belief in some people who are not at severe risk to develop COVID-19 symptoms didn't feel the need to get vaccinated.
- Some even believed that they might become ill with another disease by getting vaccinated.
- No study suggests that certain blood groups will develop more severe symptoms of COVID-19 while other blood groups will not develop very severe symptoms, yet this idea was found to be prevailing and people decided whether they require the vaccine or not [32].

Reason for Concern and Misconception Regarding the COVID-19 Vaccine in the Indian Population

Four factors can be considered as a reason for predominating myths and misconceptions of the vaccine that can be summarized as follows:

Vaccine Development in a Short Time

The very quick development of a vaccine for COVID-19 disease is the major reason for concern among health workers and others, as the first successful vaccine for SARS-COV-2 viral disease, Pfizer, was announced on 2nd December 2020, which was within a year of COVID-19 spread. Before this, the fastest vaccine, from viral sampling to approval, took 4 years to develop for mumps disease in 1960 [33].

After Pfizer, several vaccines for COVID-19 were developed in several countries around the world, including India.

The reason for the quick development of the vaccine is the advancement in technology with which it is made in a short time without compromising on safety. A large number of tests of the COVID-19 vaccine are done in a short time through the participation of a large number of people who volunteered for it. New ways of making vaccine, such as by use of mRNA, has been validated by the COVID-19 response, says Dan Barouch, director of the Center for Virology and Vaccine Research at Harvard Medical School in Boston, Massachusetts [33]. Hence, it is completely wrong to think that vaccines which are developed in a short time aren't safe to use.

Social Media Platforms Spreading Rumours About The Vaccine

With the increased use of the internet, social media has become the largest platform through which most information is disseminated swiftly nowadays. But unfortunately, this manifesto is being utilized more for spreading rumours and fake messages than using it for a good cause. Facebook, Twitter, and WhatsApp are the main platforms on which several fake messages run, and it becomes hard to identify the correct information from the wrong ones. The view-seekers in these media try to make new content, even if it is false or fake, to get more and more views for themselves.

Misconceptions or myths about the COVID-19 vaccine also is largely circulated among the population through these programs. The Director-General of WHO has warned of the potential danger of 'misinformation'. He also stressed fighting against the 'infodemic' alongside the COVID-19 pandemic. The Government of India has ordered strict action and punishment under the Disaster Management Act and the Indian Penal Code, against those spreading misinformation/rumour about the efficacy of the COVID-19 vaccine [34].

Illiteracy

Illiteracy has always remained a problem and barrier to the smooth acceptance of anything around the world including India. Several studies conducted showed that literate people took COVID-19 disease prevention norms more seriously and properly than illiterate ones [35]. 287 million people in India are illiterate, according to the 2011 census, which is fairly a great number, and educating them about the safety and benefits of the vaccine is a difficult job.

Distrust of People in the Health System

Though the health system of India has remained a backbone to fight against the SARS-CoV-2 virus disease, there is a large section of people who don't trust the distribution process of the COVID-19 vaccine, as can be seen in Fig. (**5**) of our survey, which some of the respondents have answered that they doubt on the distribution process of the vaccine.

CONCLUSION

The COVID-19 pandemic has shaken the globe on a massive scale. Scientists from all around the globe have developed various vaccines that may reduce the severity of the disease. Curiosity, safety concerns, and a lack of proper vaccine management are all deterring individuals from getting vaccinated. This questionnaire survey shed light on crucial aspects related to the vaccination process, primarily targeting the Indian population. The Indian sub-continent inhabiting 1.38 billion people, was drastically affected by the pandemic, and the Government of India had to launch a proper vaccination campaign called a "Co-WIN vaccine delivery management system". This well-managed system succeeded in vaccinating 23.44% (32.7 crores) of the Indian population in just 10 months [36]. This vaccination drive met with various myths and misconceptions owing to various reasons, as discussed briefly in the chapter. Efforts have been made to state facts and reality regarding vaccines. Thus, propagating proper awareness among people was a challenging task. There were various concerns regarding these vaccines that bug the human population resulting in a slower rate of vaccination. The chapter compiled the acceptance of the COVID-19 vaccines among the Indian population, the management system devised by the Government of India and also addresses the various myths, misconceptions and concerns that prevailed during the pandemic time, regarding the disease as well as the vaccines.

CONSENT FOR PUBLICATION

Not applicable.

CONFLICT OF INTEREST

The authors declare no conflict of interest, financial or otherwise.

ACKNOWLEDGEMENTS

The authors are thankful to Dr. (Mrs.) V. Prakash, Principal, Isabella Thoburn College, Lucknow, Integral University, Lucknow, and Era University, Lucknow, for the support.

REFERENCES

[1] Ou X, Liu Y, Lei X, *et al.* Characterization of spike glycoprotein of SARS-CoV-2 on virus entry and its immune cross-reactivity with SARS-CoV. Nat Commun 2020; 11(1): 1620. [http://dx.doi.org/10.1038/s41467-020-15562-9] [PMID: 32221306]

[2] Lai CC, Shih TP, Ko WC, Tang HJ, Hsueh PR. Severe acute respiratory syndrome coronavirus 2 (SARS-CoV-2) and coronavirus disease-2019 (COVID-19): The epidemic and the challenges. Int J Antimicrob Agents 2020; 55(3): 105924. [http://dx.doi.org/10.1016/j.ijantimicag.2020.105924] [PMID: 32081636]

[3] Lauer SA, Grantz KH, Bi Q, *et al.* The Incubation Period of Coronavirus Disease 2019 (COVID-19) From Publicly Reported Confirmed Cases: Estimation and Application. Ann Intern Med 2020; 172(9): 577-82. [http://dx.doi.org/10.7326/M20-0504] [PMID: 32150748]

[4] Yoshimoto FK. The Proteins of Severe Acute Respiratory Syndrome Coronavirus-2 (SARS CoV-2 or n-COV19), the Cause of COVID-19. Protein J 2020; 39(3): 198-216. [http://dx.doi.org/10.1007/s10930-020-09901-4] [PMID: 32447571]

[5] Silva SJR, Alves da Silva CT, Mendes RPG, Pena L. Role of nonstructural proteins in the pathogenesis of SARS-CoV-2. J Med Virol 2020; 92(9): 1427-9. [http://dx.doi.org/10.1002/jmv.25858] [PMID: 32270884]

[6] Wrapp D, Wang N, Corbett KS, *et al.* Cryo-EM structure of the 2019-nCoV spike in the prefusion conformation. Science 2020; 367(6483): 1260-3. [http://dx.doi.org/10.1126/science.abb2507] [PMID: 32075877]

[7] Jiang S, Du L, Shi Z. An emerging coronavirus causing pneumonia outbreak in Wuhan, China: calling for developing therapeutic and prophylactic strategies. Emerg Microbes Infect 2020; 9(1): 275-7. [http://dx.doi.org/10.1080/22221751.2020.1723441] [PMID: 32005086]

[8] Dhama K, Sharun K, Tiwari R, Dadar M, Malik YS, Singh KP, *et al.* COVID-19, an emerging coronavirus infection: advances and prospects in designing and developing vaccines, immunotherapeutics, and therapeutics. Hum Vaccines Immunother. 16(6):1232–8.

[9] India – COVID19 Vaccine Tracker [Internet]. [cited 2022 Jan 23]. Available from: https://covid19.trackvaccines.org/country/india/

[10] Ge H, Wang X, Yuan X, *et al.* The epidemiology and clinical information about COVID-19. Eur J Clin Microbiol Infect Dis 2020; 39(6): 1011-9. [http://dx.doi.org/10.1007/s10096-020-03874-z] [PMID: 32291542]

[11] https://peerj.com/articles/9689/

[12] https://www.sciencedirect.com/science/article/pii/S0048969720323780

[13] Chakraborty C, Agoramoorthy G. India's cost-effective COVID-19 vaccine development initiatives. Vaccine 2020; 38(50): 7883-4. [http://dx.doi.org/10.1016/j.vaccine.2020.10.056] [PMID: 33129610]

[14] https://www.bharatbiotech.com/covaxin.html

[15] https://publichealth.medresearch.in/index.php/ijphr/article/view/156

[16] Danabal KGM, Magesh SS, Saravanan S, Gopichandran V. Attitude towards COVID 19 vaccines and vaccine hesitancy in urban and rural communities in Tamil Nadu, India – a community based survey. BMC Health Serv Res 2021; 21(1): 994. [http://dx.doi.org/10.1186/s12913-021-07037-4] [PMID: 34548088]

[17] Khubchandani J, Sharma S, Price JH, Wiblishauser MJ, Webb FJ. COVID-19 Morbidity and Mortality in Social Networks: Does It Influence Vaccine Hesitancy? Int J Environ Res Public Health 2021; 18(18): 9448. [http://dx.doi.org/10.3390/ijerph18189448] [PMID: 34574373]

[18] https://indianexpress.com/article/opinion/india-has-a-vaccine-hesitancy-challenge-7388907/

[19] https://en.gaonconnection.com/covid19-rural-india-shortage-of-phc-doctors-second-wav--vaccine-hesitancy-vaccination-testing-quacks-madhya-pradesh/

[20] https://data.worldbank.org/indicator/SP.RUR.TOTL.ZS

[21] https://www.frontiersin.org/articles/10.3389/fmed.2020.585579/full

[22] https://www.aimsindia.com/blog/busting-5-myths-related-to-covid-vaccines-in-india/

[23] https://www.mohfw.gov.in/pdf/LiberalisedPricingandAcceleratedNationalCovid19VaccinationStrategy2042021.pdf

[24] Allana A. 2021.https://www.nytimes.com/2021/03/15/opinion/india-covid-vaccine.html

[25] https://economictimes.indiatimes.com/news/india/tika-utsav-indias-covid-19-vaccination-co-erage-exceeds-11-crore-mark/articleshow/82063145.cms

[26] https://www.ndtv.com/india-news/vaccinatoion-cowin-27-lakh-hits-per-minute-governmen--sources-on-vaccine-registration-2423760

[27] https://www.hindustantimes.com/india-news/200-million-vaccine-doses-administered-i--india-101621968424709.html

[28] https://indianexpress.com/article/india/in-6-months-since-launch-of-drive-vaccine-coverag--crosses-50-cr-doses-7442395/

[29] https://www.hindustantimes.com/india-news/covid19-3-states-3-uts-have-achieved-100--irst-dose-vaccination-check-list-here-101631500402671.html

[30] Perappadan BS. https://www.thehindu.com/news/national/india-administers-record-2-crore-5--lakh-covid-19-vaccine-doses-in-a-single-day-on-september-17-2021/article36512270.ece

[31] https://timesofindia.indiatimes.com/city/delhi/needle-of-suspicion-vaccine-could-lead-to--urge-in-blood-sugar-levels/articleshow/84156985.cms

[32] https://www.hopkinsmedicine.org/health/conditions-and-diseases/coronavirus/covid-19-vacc-nes-myth-versus-fact

[33] Ball P. The lightning-fast quest for COVID vaccines — and what it means for other diseases. Nature 2021; 589(7840): 16-8.
[http://dx.doi.org/10.1038/d41586-020-03626-1] [PMID: 33340018]

[34] https://www.news18.com/news/india/covid-19-coronavirus-vaccine-rumours-disaster-mana-ement-act-jail-ipc-3338240.html

[35] https://www.epw.in/engage/article/literacy-and-response-covid-19

[36] https://ourworldindata.org/covid-vaccinations

SUBJECT INDEX

A

B

C

Alfred J. Lawrence & Tahmeena Khan (Eds.)

D

E

F

G

H

I

L

M

N

O

P

R

S

T

V

Made in the USA
Las Vegas, NV
03 November 2026

57422841R00117